CNA Study Guide 2025-2026

Complete Review + 560 Questions and Detailed Answer Explanations for the Certified Nursing Assistant Exam (8 Full-Length Exams)

Table of Contents

Introduction

Certified nurse assistants have an important role in the healthcare setting. From hospital wards to resident homes, they occupy a significant position in the delivery and execution of healthcare plans. The Certified Nurse Assistant exam certifies that an individual has the required level of knowledge and skill to function in this capacity.

This guide has been put together to help candidates prepare for the CNA exam. It includes a thorough discussion of key concepts, as well as a comprehensive practice test section.

How to use this guide

- Establish a particular time for study.
- Allot some time to study the theory section and another block of time to answer the test questions.
- Try to simulate a quiet, time-restricted environment when you take the practice tests.

About the Exam

The coordination and administration of the Certified Nurse Assistant exams are usually managed by individual state nursing boards or designated testing organizations. To see if you are in one of the many NCSBN jurisdictions that recognize the CNA exam, visit https://www.ncsbn.org/.

The exam is divided into two parts, both of which must be passed to obtain the CNA certification.

- Written/oral section.
- Skills demonstration section.

The structure and content of the CNA written exam can vary significantly between states and testing agencies. The number of questions, the inclusion of non-scored items, and the specific format (such as the addition of reading comprehension questions) are not universally standardized and may differ from the description provided. The details of the exam, including the number of questions and their types, should be verified based on the specific requirements of the state or testing agency administering the exam.

Written/Oral Test

Both written and oral exams test three major domains:

- Physical care skills.
- Psychosocial care skills.
- Role of the nurse aide.

The time allotted for the written/oral test is two hours.

Skills Test

This section of the exam tests five key skills. The time allowed for the Skills Test section of the CNA exam can vary depending on the state and the testing agency. Usually, the Skills Test may take longer than 30 minutes, as candidates are required to demonstrate several skills in a realistic healthcare setting. The exact time should be verified based on the specific requirements of the state or testing agency administering the exam.

Exam registration and eligibility

Candidates are required to register on Credentia and select the state where they plan to practice. Candidates must complete a CNA training program approved by their state to be eligible for the exam.

Candidates should select the date they wish to take the exam and then pay the necessary fees. Exam fees vary from state to state. The general average is $100. Candidates who take the exam online are advised to read about the onboarding procedure before test day to avoid any glitches.

Results

The exams are reported as either passed or failed. For the skills demonstration, the score report shows if a candidate's performance was satisfactory or unsatisfactory. A satisfactory rating must be achieved in all five skills to pass this section of the test.

Exam reports are sent either by email a few hours after the exam or mailed physically to a candidate's address within five to seven business days.

Chapter 1: Role of the Nurse Aide

CNAs are healthcare workers trained to assist nurses. They understand the basic principles of nursing and are trained to help meet the basic needs of patients.

Personal Responsibility

CNAs have a personal responsibility to both the patient and other healthcare personnel.

Reporting Requirements

Reporting involves oral communication between healthcare providers about whatever care has been provided to a patient and/or the patient's status. Documentation is a written or legal record of a patient's care. This may include charts about vitals, documentation about procedures performed, and notes about medications that have been administered.

- **Chain of command**

CNAs may report directly to a nurse manager or a head nurse without as many intermediate levels. The exact chain of command should be verified based on the organizational structure of the specific healthcare facility. CNAs must know when to report to the staff nurse and when to escalate.

The elements of the reports must be kept confidential based on strict healthcare laws.

- **Legal obligation to report**

Documentation and reports may be used in medicolegal cases where there are debates about a patient's care. It is vital to report and document for every patient.

- **Elements of reports**

The elements of the reports may change based on the patient. The important elements may include any physical changes or behavioral changes in the patient. Foul odors, such as from urine, the mouth, or wounds, should be reported. Difficulty with breathing, pain in any part of the body, wounds, and wound care should also be reported.

Elements of a report may be objective or subjective. Signs (objective information) are measured by the healthcare professional. They may include temperature and pulse rate. Symptoms are subjective information given by the patient, such as complaints of chest pain or a headache. Both objective and subjective information is reported by the CNA. Objective information includes measurable signs like temperature and pulse rate, while subjective information includes symptoms described by the patient, like pain or discomfort. The CNA's role involves accurately reporting both types of information. It is also important to record and report the time accurately.

Documentation serves as a record of a patient's level of consciousness, vital signs, food intake, urine output, intravenous fluid infusions, height, weight, and response to treatment.

- **Legality of documentation**

Documentation/charts are legal documents that can be used in a court of law. This is why CNAs must write legibly, accurately, and honestly.

- **Abbreviations**

Some common abbreviations used in healthcare and medical practice include ABG (arterial blood gas), AMA (against medical advice), ALL (acute lymphoblastic leukemia), IDDM (insulin-dependent diabetes mellitus), PE (pulmonary embolism), bd (twice a day), BMR (basal metabolic rate), and CAD (coronary artery disease). Many abbreviations are standard and widely understood in the medical community. However, CNAs and other healthcare professionals should be familiar with their facility's policy regarding acceptable abbreviations and ensure that any abbreviations used are clear and unambiguous to avoid misinterpretation.

Promotion of Personal Health and Safety

The safety of patients and other healthcare workers is a priority. Though it is important to oversee the health of others, CNAs must care for themselves first.

- **Principles of body mechanics**

CNAs bend, lift, and pull a lot, so they need proper body mechanics to avoid injury to themselves and others. Body mechanics are one way to promote personal health and safety. They involve knowledge of how the body works and how to move it most safely and effectively.

There are eight fundamental principles of body mechanics:

- **Maintain proper alignment**: Body mechanics teach people to maintain the body in the right position. For instance, when upright, all the joints should be aligned. When seated, a person should keep their feet flat on the floor and their back straight.

- **Bend at the hips and knees**: When a heavy object is to be lifted, a person should bend at the hips and knees while the back is kept straight.

- **The object should be kept close to the body**: When a person lifts or carries, the object should not be held far from the body. This will limit the force exerted.

- **Use the leg muscles**: The muscles of the legs are more powerful than those of the back. It is important to use them when heavy loads are lifted and carried.

- **Avoid repetitive movements**: It is common to make repetitive motions when objects are lifted. This can put a strain on the muscles and cause damage to not only the muscles but also the tendons.

- **Use the proper equipment**: Certain equipment makes it easier and safer to lift heavy loads and reduce the stress and strain on the muscles.

- **Good posture:** Some postures can cause back problems with the back when objects are lifted.

- **Use the core muscles**: The core muscles help to keep the backbone in place and help with correct posture. A person should engage their core muscles when heavy loads are lifted or carried.

- **Injury prevention**

Injury prevention is another very important part of health and safety. One way to prevent injuries is to lift patients/loads with another person or use lifting equipment that the CNA is trained to use.

- **Self-care**

The work of a CNA can be demanding. This can cause a lot of stress physically and mentally. Research has shown that self-care is important to help maintain a CNA's health. This includes good sleep habits, exercise, and a balanced diet.

Promotion and Protection of Patient Rights

CNAs must be aware of patient rights, which are protected and enforced by federal regulations.

Some of these rights include:

- Patients have the legal right not to be pressured, discriminated against, or punished by a healthcare facility. They are entitled to the best care available and have the right to choose the type of care they receive. This includes informed consent, which means a person's right to be in control of what happens to their body.
- Patients need to know their rights and what services are available to them.
- Patients are entitled to choose their doctors, caregivers, and treatments.
- The Health Insurance Portability and Accountability Act of 1996 (HIPAA) protects patients' right to private, unsupervised communication with whomever they choose.
- Patients deserve dignity, respect, and freedom.
- Patients are entitled to remain in a facility unless a transfer or discharge is necessary. Any changes to the location must be made in a safe manner and with the knowledge and consent of the patient.
- Patients' personal property must remain secure at all times and may not be removed or used without consent.
- Patients are entitled to freedom from any kind of physical or mental restrictions, as well as from any psychoactive drugs used for disciplinary rather than medical reasons.

It is the responsibility of CNAs to recognize and report violations of these patient rights to the appropriate person in the chain of command.

Patient abuse may be psychological, physical, financial, neglectful, or sexual. Physical abuse may be evidenced by physical injuries on the hands, feet, neck, and other body parts. Psychological abuse may be indicated by depression, cognitive decline, and memory deficits. Financial abuse in the healthcare context refers to the illegal or improper use of a patient's funds, property, or assets. This can include stealing money or belongings, forging signatures, or coercing patients into financial transactions or changes in wills or trusts. A switch of healthcare facilities, from hospitals to nursing homes, does not constitute financial abuse in itself, unless it is done for the financial benefit of the caregiver or institution against the patient's will or best interests.

Staff and members of the healthcare team should be properly trained on how to identify and report abuse. One key risk factor for patient abuse is staff burnout or stress. CNAs and other healthcare workers may be overworked and direct hostility toward patients.

To better promote and protect the rights of their patients, CNAs must understand diversity, which includes gender, sex, class, culture, education, and religion. Different cultural perspectives determine the attitudes of both CNAs and patients.

Another aspect of the promotion and protection of the rights of patients is to understand how to resolve grievances. A conflict is a serious disagreement in which two or more perspectives, needs, or motivations are incompatible with one another. When the conflict is expressed in public, it can result in confrontations between the parties.

Here are a few strategies to settle grievances among patients and other healthcare workers:

- Stay calm and collected.
- Ask a manager or a mediator for help.
- Find a quiet spot away from colleagues, patients, or their families.
- Listen to both sides.

A patient's rights also involve care given to the patient's personal belongings. This includes hearing aids, glasses, jewelry, medications, dentures, prosthetics, phones, tablets, assistive devices, wallets, handbags, keys, or clothing. Hospital management should provide a secure environment where a patient's property can be locked up.

Time Management and Work Prioritization

A CNA must be able to prioritize and effectively manage time. Here are a few strategies for time management:

- **Planning**: Planning helps to classify projects into emergency and urgent. Emergency projects are prioritized, and non-urgent work can be postponed.

- To increase time efficiency, CNAs can write down all information, take notes, and take vitals between charting periods. For many, the busiest part of the day is around patients' mealtimes, as the majority of patients receive services at that time. Therefore, CNAs must plan for this.

- Delegation can help improve efficiency.

- Avoid multitasking. Research has demonstrated that this practice is not productive, contrary to popular belief. This is because the division of attention leads to a decrease in cognitive resources and productivity.

- Eliminate distractions. Interruptions are unavoidable. However, if you need to focus on an important task, politely request that you not be interrupted unless it's urgent.

- Catch up on low-priority tasks during downtime.

- Take breaks. Attempts to just "push through" work without a single break can lead to exhaustion and reduced productivity.

Workplace Standards

CNAs must be cognizant of their ethical responsibilities in the medical profession. Violation of a patient's rights, such as privacy, autonomy, expression of opinion, and other human rights, is subject to disciplinary action.

Unacceptable actions in the workplace include:

- The use of a personal phone in a patient care area.

- Failure to respond promptly to call lights when available.

- Failure to answer assigned phone(s).

- The use of agency computers for private purposes.

- Avoidance of clients due to their ethnicity, religion, demeanor, or other characteristics.

- Solicitation and/or acceptance of gifts or other gratuities from patients and their families.

CNA Registry

CNAs should verify the specific registration requirements in their state, and if there is a registry. The information in the registry includes things like a person's training, criminal history, skills, and if they've been found guilty of abuse, neglect, or other disciplinary issues. Some states won't let healthcare providers hire someone if they've been convicted of certain crimes.

Certifications vary based on the state and the employer. In most cases, CNAs will need to renew their certification every year or two. The exact renewal process varies from state to state. CNAs need to pay a fee and provide proof of continuing education credits. In addition, skills such as CPR need to be recertified every two years.

Before a CNA is hired, an employer will perform a criminal background check to determine if the individual has a criminal record. If so, the employer may look for a waiver to allow them to work.

CNAs as Members of the Healthcare Team

CNAs are required to complete at least 75 hours of training, divided into classroom instruction hours and clinical hours. In addition, they must have valid certifications and pass a state board of certifications exam.

CNA Job Responsibilities

CNAs assist with the basics of patient healthcare, including baths, walks, meals, and other activities of daily living. They may also help move patients from beds to chairs and keep rooms stocked. In some settings, CNAs may have additional duties, such as assisting with certain medical procedures under supervision or providing more specialized care to patients with specific needs.

CNAs must assist within the limits of their educational and certification qualifications. They may not exceed their certification levels, as this exposes them and the healthcare facility to legal liability in the event of a patient-related incident.

Interdisciplinary Team Member Roles

Some of the other members within a healthcare community include doctors, nurses, therapists (occupational, respiratory, speech and physical, etc.), dietitians, and nutritionists. Every member of the team has received specific training for their role.

Doctors diagnose patients and make treatment decisions. Nurses interpret orders from doctors, follow orders, conduct patient evaluations, and perform nursing interventions.

Teamwork Principles

CNAs need to be able to collaborate with all team members to provide the highest quality of care. They must be respectful and stay on schedule and on task. It is important to know when to notify someone when there's a change in patient status and whom to report it to.

Collaboration is defined as the process of two or more people working together to create or produce something. It can take place in person or online.

Some principles of effective teamwork include:

- **Trust**: People need a safe space to share and receive feedback, to be motivated by a shared purpose, and to have the resources and support they need to connect. All of this can only be achieved in an environment of trust, where employees have the best interests of their colleagues and leaders in mind.
- **Empathy:** Every member of the team, as well as patients, has different challenges, so an empathetic approach is important.
- **Accountability**: Every member of a team needs to be accountable to each other.

The Care Planning Process and Implementation

CNAs assist with the implementation of patient care plans. CNAs contribute valuable observations and feedback based on their direct care experiences, which can inform the ongoing evaluation and adjustment of care plans. These plans are evaluated for their effectiveness and changed as needed (e.g., based on a patient's response).

The five-step process to plan nursing care includes:

- **Assessment**: The nurse gathers facts and information about the patient. This includes the vital signs, history of the illness, and other facts important for a diagnosis.
- **Diagnosis**: Based on the facts collected from a patient, the healthcare team arrives at a diagnosis, which determines the modality of treatment.
- **Outcomes and planning**: The healthcare team comes up with goals that must be achieved in the treatment of the patient. This may be subject to the patient's condition and the stage of the disease.
- **Implementation**: The goals that have been set forth by the team are implemented.
- **Evaluation**: Scales and guidelines may be used in this final step of the nursing care plan to ensure the goals set for a patient have been met.

CNAs' Responsibility to Provide Care Per the Care Plan

Once the nursing care plan has been established by the nurse, CNAs must provide care based on that plan. For example, they may need to evaluate patients to determine if they need to be turned to avoid skin problems, provide regular care to the perineal area, and make sure the patient gets meal trays.

Interpersonal Relations or Communication Skills

CNAs need to be great communicators. They should be able to take care of a patient but also be able to talk to other healthcare professionals and ensure the patient gets the best care possible.

Communication Principles

In a healthcare community, there will always be different levels of communication required. These include basic messages received at the start of a shift and the communication of potential problems and issues to those next in the chain of command.

CNAs need to be honest and open when they communicate with patients. They must ensure their approach is both professional and empathetic. Although it is important for CNAs not to make patients feel uncomfortable, they should provide necessary information and guidance relevant to the patient's care and wellbeing. However, CNAs should avoid giving personal opinions or medical advice that falls outside their scope of practice. They should focus on factual information related to the care they are providing and refer to the nurse or physician for more detailed medical information or advice.

There are seven major principles of communication:

- **Clarity**: The message from the sender to the receiver should be clear. The words and tone must be unambiguous. The receiver must understand whatever the sender says.

- **Attention**: People have different attention spans, so it can be difficult for CNAs to get the attention of some patients.

- **Feedback**: Feedback helps the sender of the message to know whether the receiver got the message, understood it, and will now act on the message. Feedback may be verbal, written, or audiovisual.

- **Informality**: Not all patients are the same. Sometimes informal communication is better. For instance, a resident who does not understand why a procedure should be done might only need a simple conversation.

- **Consistency**: Communication should be consistent with what the team stands for and the patient's decisions.

- **Timeliness**: Information should be conveyed on time. For example, a patient who is supposed to have surgery should be informed days before the procedure and consent should be taken.

- **Adequacy**: Communication needs to be accurate and complete in all aspects. Proper information is necessary to make correct decisions and action plans.

Communication Types

There are three main types of communication: **written, nonverbal,** and **verbal.** Verbal communication takes place naturally when people talk to each other. This includes face-to-face communication as well as phone calls.

Information is transmitted through written, electronic (text, fax, email, etc.), and nonverbal communication (body language and facial expressions).

Other forms of communication include:

- **Visual communication**: This form of communication may not be so common in the workplace. It includes things like video chats.
- **Listening**: Active listening is probably the most important communication type. You have to do more than just hear a person's words. You have to listen to the real message behind them. This is vital in a healthcare setting.

Factors that Affect Communication

Communication is the foundation of the healthcare team's success. To maintain good communication, there are several factors to consider.

- **Language barriers and cultural diversity**: Do the speakers speak (and understand) the same language? Communities are becoming increasingly diverse and multilingual. Different languages can quickly lead to communication issues. This will require help from a translator. A family member can also come in and help from time to time. Cultural differences can affect how someone speaks.
- **Nonverbal barriers**: It is essential for CNAs not to create additional nonverbal boundaries. For example, patients may not be comfortable with a medical professional who holds a phone in their hand as it may appear as though the CNA is disinterested, which can impede effective communication.
- **Physical barriers**: Physical impediments to communication may exist. These may include sensory impairments, such as hearing, vision, speech, or sensory impairments. Patients may have cognitive impairments that impede their ability to comprehend or communicate.

Therapeutic Communication Techniques

Therapeutic communication may be necessary to bridge the communication and collaboration gaps between CNAs and their patients.

- CNAs should use caution when sharing personal experiences or indicating that they have gone through a similar situation as the patient. While empathetic understanding is important, self-disclosure must be professional and focused on the patient's needs rather than the CNA's personal experiences. The primary goal of therapeutic communication is to understand and address the patient's feelings and concerns, not to share or compare personal stories. This approach ensures that the conversation remains patient-centered and professional.

- CNAs can also ask patients to share their thoughts or point out a common theme to help improve communication.
- Dialogue with patients and inquiries about the particular events that have caused them distress are effective methods of inquiry.
- Questions about how someone feels can be a great way to start a conversation. CNAs should show appreciation and make sure patients feel important and taken care of. This can also help with communication. Of course, everyone is different, so what works with one patient might not work with another.

All of these are therapeutic communication skills that are important for CNAs.

Chapter 2: Promotion of Safety

Potential Hazards in Healthcare Environments

Healthcare workers, especially CNAs, are exposed to potential hazards within the healthcare facility. These hazards are grouped into different categories based on their severity. They include hospital-acquired infections, exposure to chemicals, toxic waste, radiation, and psychological problems.

Some of these potential hazards are discussed below.

Infections

Healthcare providers are expected to be aware of safety measures to avoid the spread of infectious diseases such as Hepatitis A, B, C, tuberculosis, HIV/AIDS, and other viral diseases (measles, influenza, etc.). The major mode of transmission of infectious diseases is by direct contact with sources of the virus, such as blood, saliva, semen, or other body fluids.

CNAs and other healthcare providers are at risk of infection by needles, exposure to body fluids, and by not following the standard hygiene procedures.

Measures to prevent infections include:

- Disinfection.
- Use of personal protective equipment (PPE).
- Handwashing practices.
- Sensitization and education of the public on safe measures.
- Vaccination.
- Use of face masks.
- Adequate ventilation.
- Patient isolation for individuals with communicable diseases.

CNAs should follow standard precautions with all patients to prevent the spread of infection and be aware of the infection control policies of their healthcare facility.

Exposure to Chemicals and Toxic Waste

Certain chemicals can lead to genetic mutations, cancer, allergies, hair loss, and other adverse effects.

Cytotoxic drugs are hazardous and irritate the skin and eyes. For instance, formalin, a chemical that is used to preserve organs, and ethylene oxide, used for sterilization of medical instruments, are both commonly found in surgical suites, dialysis rooms, and other clinical areas. These chemicals contain carcinogenic agents and can be linked to the onset of respiratory, nervous, and integumentary complications.

CNAs and other medical workers should be educated on how to handle chemicals to avoid spills and protect themselves and patients from adverse effects.

Radiation

CNAs may be present in environments where radiography is performed, but their exposure is typically minimal and well within safety guidelines due to protective measures. Healthcare providers are mandated to protect themselves within the guidelines of their state.

Psychological Problems

Psychological problems that occur in the healthcare facility can be attributed to emotional and mental distress on the job. Often, these circumstances revolve around work ethics and physical demands. For example, CNAs are exposed to assault and injury, especially in psychiatric, pediatric, and emergency units.

There is also the issue of heavy workloads. Sometimes, CNAs have to run shifts continuously over a period of time and might not have the time to see their loved ones. This impacts attitude and behavior, which can lead to decreased job performance and absenteeism.

Stress management for CNAs often involves self-care strategies, seeking support from supervisors, and utilizing available resources within the healthcare facility. To prevent violence, preventive measures such as adequate security, education of patients and healthcare workers, and legal structures should be implemented.

It is important to understand the impact of hazards within the hospital environment on healthcare providers and patients. This allows medical professionals to adopt safe techniques to either prevent or control the risks.

Common Patient Injuries

Skin tears occur when there is a break in the skin. The skin layer can be partially removed or totally lifted. Skin tears can result from trauma or blunt force, a cut or scrape (known as shearing), or friction that results when the skin is rubbed.

In nursing homes, skin tears are common wounds that elderly people have to deal with because of the increased risk of falls, immobility, and chronic illnesses common among this age group. When skin tears or other minor injuries happen, they should normally heal in a few days. However, they can progress into chronic wounds. Patients may develop chronic wounds as a result of diseases, repeated falls, friction, burns, bruises, pressure areas, and hospital-acquired infections.

CNAs play a role in implementing strategies to reduce or prevent the risk of skin tears. CNAs contribute by following established protocols and guidelines for skin care and by providing direct patient care under supervision. These tears affect the epidermis and dermis, which can cause deep wounds on the hands, legs, and other parts of the upper and lower limbs. CNAs are required to assess skin integrity and document and report patients' medical history to other healthcare providers.

Elderly individuals have less collagen, which leads to less skin elasticity and wrinkles. Their skin begins to dry out, and there is a constriction of blood vessels, which affects the blood supply to the skin and limbs. Therefore, the skin is vulnerable. Bandages might damage the skin and lead to worsened tears.

CNAs are expected to establish patient-centered care to improve skin health.

To manage common injuries, CNAs should:

- Observe skin changes in the elderly and inform the nurse or doctor.
- Encourage and monitor skin hygiene in patients. This includes bed baths, skin hygiene, urinary catheters, etc.
- Care for patients with mobility impairments and wound dressings.
- Reposition unconscious or immobile patients to prevent pressure areas.
- Incorporate daily exercise routines to improve blood circulation.
- Educate patients on safety measures within and outside the healthcare facility.

CNAs should understand the basic functions of the integumentary system and follow sterile principles to address infections. CNAs are responsible for adhering to established protocols and procedures in their daily work. They should also be able to tell when signs and symptoms of unhealthy skin conditions appear and escalate to the appropriate healthcare professional as necessary.

Risks Related to Common Injuries

Severe injuries predispose patients to the risk of internal hemorrhage, fractures, hematoma, dislocation, and skin sores, which occur mostly with falls or accidents that affect the aged.

Osteoporosis in the elderly affects bone density and strength, leading to an increased risk of fractures, particularly from falls. It's the reduced bone density associated with osteoporosis that particularly increases the risk of fractures. CNAs should be aware of these risks and assist with mobility and activities that prevent falls. CNAs should monitor patient baths and provide assistance with mobility.

CNAs must use proper posture when they lift heavy loads. They should also know when to ask for help or use lifting equipment.

Safety and Comfort

Comfort of the Patients

The physical aspects of comfort provision seek to protect patients from pain and hazards, while the emotional aspect covers protection from anxiety or depression.

To provide patients with comfort, CNAs should:

- Participate fully in nursing care.
- Monitor patients.
- Listen and talk to patients.
- Use a warm touch to help patients relax.
- Be aware of the importance of patient positioning.
- Employ hygienic practices.
- Adapt the environment to suit the specific needs of patients.
- Provide the right diet to patients at the right time.
- Assist patients with sleep needs.
- Assist patients with the elimination of waste.

CNAs should ensure patient comfort throughout the entire care process, including during and after procedures. This involves being attentive to the patient's physical and emotional needs, employing proper techniques to alleviate pain or discomfort, and making adjustments to improve the patient's overall comfort. It is associated with rest, exercise, and the adjustment of the patient's body to the bed and the environment.

Devices can be used to add comfort, relieve discomfort, and help maintain correct posture. These devices include pillows, bed cradles, air and water mattresses, foot and knee rests, bed blocks, etc.

Accident Prevention

CNAs are expected to predict an individual's risk of injuries based on a clinical assessment of the history of falls, the cause and its severity, loss of consciousness and dizziness associated with underlying causes, reduced pace while walking, and other disruptions of mobility. A fall assessment involves a detailed history of patients, questions about their muscular functions, and assessment of edema, weakness, and anxiety disorders.

A patient with a high risk for falls should have a bed with rails and be provided with assistance at mealtimes, especially if the client has frequent tremors. Assisted baths should also be implemented.

Patients who have had a previous history of falls are at high risk. This applies to patients with neurological disorders, musculoskeletal dysfunction, and cardiovascular diseases.

Restraint Techniques and Alternatives

Restraint techniques are physical strategies implemented to keep an individual in a position for some time. This means that the upper and lower limbs or other body parts are limited from movement with belts, straps, bedrails, etc.

Although restraints may be used in psychiatric settings as a last resort to prevent harm to the patient or others, the use of restraints is highly regulated and should only be employed when absolutely necessary and under strict guidelines. The decision to use restraints, particularly in combination with medications, is made by qualified healthcare professionals and is based on a thorough assessment of the patient's condition.

However, restraints can worsen the situation and cause emotional and physical damage, such as depression, confusion or bruises, edema, and other injuries. The use of restraints can lead to an increased risk of injury, agitation, and physical complications like pressure ulcers and muscle atrophy.

Therefore, restriction alternatives should be adopted by CNAs. These include:

- Flexible, patient-centered routines.
- Reassessment of patients with cognitive impairment.
- Monitored medications.
- Alternatives to restraints based on the care facility's guidelines.
- Use of professional restraint fading techniques.
- Observation of behavioral triggers in patients and facilitation of distractions, such as TV, games, exercise, etc.
- Monitor patients in nursing homes and engage them in discussions to reduce aggressive reactions.
- Teamwork among all professionals in the hospital to discuss strategies for assessment and total client care (drug dosage, intake and output, need for restraints, and types of restrictions to implement).

Legal Implications in the Use of Restraints

The use of restraints depends on legal, informative, cultural, and environmental factors.

Patients who are restrained for too long begin to feel neglected, traumatized, and hopeless, and this affects their autonomy, self-esteem, self-actualization, and self-respect. Thus, the use of restraints can lead to legal actions by the client or relatives.

For example, when chemical restraints are given in the form of medications and side effects are not explained and documented along with informed consent obtained, this could result in legal implications.

CNAs should apply the following guidelines to avoid legal issues when restraints are used on patients:

- Perform and document patient assessment for risk of injuries.
- Collaborate with healthcare providers on alternatives to care and restraints.
- For emergency cases, all restraints used must be documented.
- Outcomes of the use of restraints, which include side effects, alternatives, benefits, coping mechanisms, etc., must be documented and explained to the patients' relatives.

- The patient's preferences and consent are important, but the decision to use restraints, particularly medication, is based on a clinical assessment and the healthcare provider's judgment. Informed consent should be obtained whenever possible, and all uses of restraints should be documented thoroughly.

Risk Factors for Elopement

There are risk factors that can lead to elopement, which must be prevented by CNAs. Some of these include:

- **Neurological disorders**

This is associated with nervous breakdown, delirium, dementia, and other cognitive disorders that are common in the aged.

- **Effects of medications**

Some medications including certain types of antidepressants can cause side effects like agitation or restlessness. CNAs and healthcare professionals monitor patients on these medications for a variety of side effects.

- **Insufficient patient supervision**

CNAs have a lot of critical conditions to manage. However, with task delegation and security systems, patient elopement can be mitigated.

- **Medical history of mental disorders**

Patients with a history of mental disorders at any point in their lives should be monitored for risk of elopement.

- **Patients without mobility issues**

These patients can go on short walks and use the bathrooms with little or no supervision. Patients without mobility issues generally require less supervision for routine activities like short walks or using the bathroom, and the primary reason for monitoring them is mainly to ensure their safety and provide assistance if needed.

- **Inadequate security**

When facilities are not properly secured, it is very easy for patients to leave unnoticed.

- **Emotional and physical distress**

Depression, isolation, threats of violence by other patients, anxiety, etc., can lead to patients' elopement because they do not feel safe. Also, lifestyle changes, unmet needs, and difficulty adjusting can lead to elopement.

A lack of education on how to monitor patients can cause a huge problem for nursing homes. This means strategies to assess patients at risk for elopement and environmental modifications, such as improved security systems. Tags, color codes, and strict monitoring should be put in place.

Patients should be assessed from time to time to check behavioral or physical changes that can put them at risk of elopement from the care facility.

Safety Devices

Safety devices are important to protect patients and ensure their well-being.

These devices include:

- **Emergency alerts**

Emergency alerts are call buttons installed in areas accessible to patients (bedside, bathrooms, and common rooms). They also include fire or smoke alarms. These alarms are audible and can be used to alert medical personnel in cases of medical emergencies, such as falls, cardiovascular attacks, injuries, etc.

- **Wander guards**

Wander guards are electronic devices that beep when patients wander into hazardous areas. Staff are alerted and can provide prompt intervention to ensure the safety of patients. These devices are commonly used for patients with cognitive disorders (Alzheimer's disease, delirium, dementia, or sudden onset of confusion and disorientation).

- **Bedrails, bed, and chair alarms**

Bedrails can help to prevent patients from rolling out of bed, but they also pose a risk of entrapment and are not suitable for all patients. Chair alarms alert staff when a patient tries to stand up, indicating the potential for a fall, but they do not prevent the fall from occurring.

- **Video surveillance cameras**

Video surveillance cameras monitor patients' safety and can provide evidence if an incident occurs.

- **Patient-monitoring centers**

These centers have alarm systems that can help CNAs identify patients who have fallen.

- **Entry supervision systems**

Entry supervision systems are placed in common areas where essential care is given (medication supply rooms, sterile areas, health records) to control who has access. This ensures that only approved medical personnel or staff can access such rooms.

Infection Prevention and Control

Maintain a Clean Environment

A clean hospital environment reduces the spread of infections, promotes health, enhances comfort, and improves the safety and wellness of patients. The basics of a hygienic care environment include:

- Regularly clean surfaces that can be touched, such as side tables, beds and handrails, doorknobs, and buttons.
- Disinfect baths and toilets.
- Dispose of waste, such as syringes, soiled dressings, etc.
- Monitor routine cleaning of rooms and common areas.
- Ensure that dirty clothing is washed regularly.
- Regularly train CNAs and care providers on updated infection control techniques to maintain a clean environment and prevent infections.
- Educate patients and relatives on hygienic practices during and after hospital visits.

Factors that Contribute to the Spread of Disease-causing Organisms

Diseases are spread by microorganisms (pathogens, bacteria, viruses, fungi, etc.) due to these factors:

- **Airborne pathogens**: These microorganisms facilitate the spread of diseases through the air.
- **Disease vectors (mosquitoes, tsetse fly, parasitic worms)**: These disease agents' operations are highly dependent on the conditions of the environment.
- **Poor hygienic practices**: Bad practices can cause the spread of diseases. For example, improper disposal of waste, unhygienic preparation of meals, unclean water, exposure to disease-causing organisms, etc. In situations where patients with contagious diseases are not isolated from others and handwashing practices are not implemented, all these can predispose patients to diseases.
- Lack of adherence to health guidelines such as vaccination, use of face masks, sterilization, disinfection, handwashing, use of gloves before contact with bodily fluids, etc., can cause the spread of disease.
- **Antibiotic resistance**: Antibiotic resistance occurs when bacteria become resistant to the antibiotics that are designed to kill them. This resistance usually develops due to the overuse or misuse of antibiotics, which can cause bacteria to evolve in ways that render these drugs less effective or ineffective.
- **Environmental factors**: These include proximity to regions like wildlife habitats, tropical areas, etc., which affects the distribution of disease vectors. For example, tropical areas are known for the abundance of mosquitoes, which can lead to malaria.

Also, climatic conditions can influence the prevalence of certain microorganisms that cause diseases.

- **Geographical factors**: These include overpopulation and underpopulation, which can predispose individuals to the rapid spread of diseases.
- **Lack of access to standard healthcare facilities**: This also includes a lack of infrastructures that can detect and prevent the spread of infections.

Signs and Symptoms of Infections

Infections can present in a variety of ways, with moderate to severe symptoms.

Infections frequently show the following symptoms:

- **Fever**: A raised body temperature is among the most prevalent symptoms of an infection. This is part of the body's natural defense against infection, which helps to boost the immune system.

- **Pain**: Infections frequently cause both localized and widespread pain. This may present as a sore throat, earache, abdominal pain, joint and muscle pain, etc.
- **Sweating and chills**: Sudden sweats and chills are major indications of fever, which can be symptoms of many infectious diseases.
- **Fatigue**: A common sign of infections is feeling abnormally weak or dehydrated. This is because a person feels exhausted as their body diverts energy to combat the invasive microorganisms.
- **Cough**: A chronic cough is a common symptom of respiratory infections such as the flu, the common cold, and pneumonia.
- **Shortness of breath**: Serious lung or respiratory infections may make breathing difficult.
- **Nausea, bowel discomfort, and vomiting**: Infections of the gastrointestinal tract can cause nausea and vomiting in addition to diarrhea and stomach pain.
- **Inflammation, redness, and soreness**: Skin infections like cellulitis or abscesses can cause inflammation, redness, and soreness of the skin.
- **Rash**: Some infectious diseases, such as measles or chicken pox, result in characteristic skin rashes. Itching and redness are symptoms of other conditions, such as bacterial or fungal skin diseases.
- **Throat irritation**: Bacterial infections of the throat or viral respiratory infections can present with a painful throat.
- **Frequent urination**: Urinary tract infections (UTIs) frequently cause symptoms like frequent urination, urge to urinate, burning or pain when urinating, and blood in the urine.
- **Headache**: Numerous infections, especially infections caused by viruses, increase pressure in the head and cause headaches.
- **Discharge**: Some infections, such as STIs, can cause abnormal discharge from the vagina, anus, or mouth.
- **Confusion**: Serious neurological infections, particularly in the elderly, can confuse changes in cognitive status or agitation.

Practices that Decrease the Risk of Exposure to Disease-causing Organisms

- **Standard precautions**

Standard precautions are essential infection-control strategies designed to stop the spread of contagious diseases in healthcare environments.

These standard precautions are:

- **Handwashing**: Healthcare professionals should thoroughly wash their hands with soap and water or use a hand sanitizer that contains at least 60% alcohol before and after contact with patients, after glove removal, and whenever their hands are visibly soiled. Patients must be educated on how to wash their hands properly.
- **Prevent the spread of infectious droplets in the air**: To stop the spread of infectious droplets, both patients and healthcare professionals are expected to cover their mouth and nose with a tissue or their elbow when they cough or sneeze. Masks should be used by health workers and professionals when infections are severe.
- **Safe injection and waste disposal practices**: Used needles should never be recapped and should be disposed of immediately in a designated sharps container, not in a regular trash can. Recapping needles poses a significant risk of needlestick injuries, which can cause the transmission of bloodborne pathogens. Sharps containers are specifically designed to safely dispose of items like needles, which prevents injury and the potential spread of infections. Waste should be regularly disposed of.
- **Environmental cleaning**: Proper cleaning is essential to prevent the spread of infections.
- **Prompt disposal of dirty linens**: Prompt disposal or laundering of soiled linens is vital to prevent the spread of infections.

- **Transmission-based precautions**

Transmission-based precautions are implemented to prevent direct contact with microorganisms or vectors in healthcare environments. These precautions include:

- **Protection from contact with microorganisms**: Contact with microorganisms may be direct or indirect. Healthcare professionals can protect themselves with gloves and gowns.
- **Protection from contact with air particles**: When they care for patients with respiratory tract infections, CNAs must wear masks.

- **Personal protective equipment (PPE)**

PPE includes sterile gloves, surgical gowns, nose masks, and eye safety equipment. Healthcare workers should be trained in how to identify the right PPE to wear based on the type of patient care to be rendered.

PPE includes:

- **Gloves**: These protect the skin of healthcare professionals when they handle blood, bodily fluids, and contaminated surfaces.
- **Gowns**: Gowns protect clothes and the skin from contact with microorganisms. They are used in situations where CNAs may come into contact with chemicals, bodily fluids, or infectious materials.
- **Masks**: Masks are used to protect the wearer from infectious particles in the air.
- **Eye protection**: Goggles or face shields are used to protect the eyes from chemicals or infectious agents.
- **Foot covers**: Foot covers, or shoe covers, are primarily used in healthcare settings to maintain a clean environment, particularly in areas like operating rooms or clean rooms where sterility is paramount. The main purpose of shoe covers is to prevent the tracking of potentially infectious materials or other contaminants into clean areas.

PPE, along with compliance with standard and transmission-based precautions, is vital to reduce the risk of hospital-acquired infections. Improper or inadequate use of PPE can lead to exposure to disease-causing organisms, which puts both healthcare workers and patients at risk of life-threatening infections.

Emergencies

Emergency and Disaster Response Protocols

Emergency services are promptly rendered when there is an immediate patient burden beyond the normal. This includes trauma from accidents, violence, or self-inflicted wounds. Disasters are classified as minor, moderate, or major based on the number of people involved and the services needed. Disasters can include floods, fire outbreaks, radiation leaks, system malfunctions, etc.

The principle of triage is applied when patients are prioritized based on the care they should be given. It includes an assessment of:

- Airway.
- Bleeding problems: severe head injuries and open chest and abdominal wounds.
- Burns and severe shock.
- Spinal cord injuries and multiple fractures.

- Minor fractures and injuries.

Immediate Lifesaving Techniques

Immediate lifesaving techniques include prompt rescue operations, triage, and emergency management by a team of health personnel. For emergency resuscitation measures, CNAs must first assess the situation, make the area safe, and assess all casualties before first aid is rendered. Patients should be removed from the danger zone before assistance is rendered.

CNA also assesses casualties for breathing, circulation, and bleeding distress. CPR is initiated if necessary, followed by immediate contact with emergency services.

Evacuation Procedures

Evacuation procedures are essential to ensure the safety of patients, particularly in emergencies such as fires, natural disasters, or other crises. Evacuation procedures involve collaboration among health professionals with consideration for patients' individual needs, such as impaired mobility or neurological functions.

CNAs should be trained in how to follow emergency routes to safely lead patients out of the disaster area. CNAs should also know how to put out fires, maintain equipment used in evacuation, such as wheelchairs, stretchers, and medical supplies, and sort these supplies for easy access in emergency cases.

Fire Prevention and Safety

Fire prevention and safety is a priority for all healthcare professionals within a care facility. CNAs must identify and rule out potential hazards such as electrical appliances, kitchen equipment, and highly flammable medical equipment. Smoke detectors and fire extinguishers must be inspected regularly.

Furthermore, healthcare professionals must be consistently trained and drilled on fire prevention techniques, safety, evacuation procedures, and the use of extinguishers. Patients must also be educated regularly on the need for safety, the use of alarms, and how to respond to incidents.

Chapter 3: Promotion of Health

Health promotion encompasses a wide range of skills, assistance, and care given to patients within a healthcare facility.

The following skills are required of a CNA:

Personal Care Skills

Feeding

Patients with cognitive impairment are usually assisted with feeding. They are given enough fluids during and between meals to increase their daily fluid consumption and prevent dehydration.

Patients must be properly positioned for feeding, and caregivers should adopt effective strategies to attend to individual needs. Patients should be placed in an upright position with heads and limbs properly supported with a pillow, cushion, or stool as necessary.

Proper positioning reduces the risk of indigestion, aspiration, or choking, and CNAs should sit at the same level with patients to observe mealtimes and make observations. These observations may include a patient's inability to chew, difficulty swallowing, coughing or choking, dislike of a particular meal, or storing food in the cheeks.

CNAs should feed patients slowly and practice good hygiene before and after meals. The dietitian should be asked to help draft a meal plan, and extra-hot meals should be avoided.

Patients who can feed themselves can be monitored or assisted, and they should be encouraged to drink plenty of fluids and clean up after meals.

Baths

CNAs in care homes assist patients with baths to remove dirt, prevent pressure sores, reduce body odor, and promote the circulation of blood. Baths are necessary to help patients regain strength, promote a sense of well-being, and ensure good health. This procedure should be tailored based on individual preferences.

Patients may be given bed baths, assisted to the bathroom, assisted to use a bathtub, or monitored as they clean up in bed. This is based on individual circumstances and conditions attached to mobility. For example, an amputee or paralyzed patient will need thorough assistance with a bed bath as compared to an individual who can reach the bathroom alone.

A bed bath comprises:

- **Complete bed bath**: Here, the CNA bathes the entire body of a dependent patient in bed.
- **Self-help bed bath**: Patients who need help in bed are usually assisted to clean parts of the body their hands might not be able to reach, e.g., the back, perineal area, or feet.
- **Partial bath**: This involves body parts that can cause odor, such as the armpits, face and hair, hands, perineum, and back.

CNAs must prepare all the materials needed for a bath, such as a basin of warm water (specific to body temperature needs), soap, towels, clean clothes, bed linen, gloves, and disinfectants. For example, when a patient with AIDS or infected wounds is bathed, the CNA should use an apron or gloves.

Procedure for bed baths

- Position the bed as high as possible to prevent strain on the CNA's back.
- All windows and doors should be closed as air current increases heat loss from the body easily.
- Provide privacy to clients.
- Clean the eyes carefully from the inner corner to the outer corner.
- Clean body parts firmly from the proximal to distal regions to increase venous return.
- Wipe perineal areas dry.

When assisting patients with baths using a bathroom or tub, CNAs should ensure that the water temperature is safe and comfortable. It should ideally be around 100 to 102°F. Water temperatures of 105 to 110°F can be too hot and pose a risk of burns, especially for elderly patients or those with sensitive skin. It's important to always check the water temperature to prevent scalding. For patients who need assistance to bathe distal parts of the body, CNAs should stand by to provide such care. The door should be kept unlocked, and a shower chair can be provided if necessary. When a patient is bathing, CNAs should respect their privacy while also ensuring their safety. The frequency of checks should be based on the patient's condition and level of independence. In some cases, it might be more appropriate to remain nearby and available for assistance or to use a call system that allows the patient to alert the CNA if needed. The approach should balance the patient's privacy with their safety. A CNA should offer to dry the patient after the bath and assist with the choice of clothes and dressing.

Bathtubs should be disinfected before use. Also, the water temperature should be monitored, and patients should not be left unaided. A bathmat should be placed in front of a tub and at the entrance of a bathroom to prevent falls as a result of splashes or spills.

Perineal Care

Perineal care is the cleansing of the perineal area, i.e., the genital or anal area. This is needed for incontinent patients, bedridden individuals, and patients with an indwelling catheter.

The intent of perineal care is to prevent skin breakdown, odor, foul discharge, itching, burning, and infections. Perineal care can be performed at least once a day, and all infection-prevention principles must be applied.

CNAs must provide quality perineal care to all patients, both male and female. They should:

- Obtain informed consent from patients and explain the procedure and its importance.
- Provide patients with privacy.
- Perform hand hygiene.
- Prepare all materials that will be needed during the procedure (towels, gloves, basin of water, cotton swabs, washcloth, laundry bag).
- Maintain respect for patients throughout the procedure.

- **For female patients**

The CNA washes her hands, gathers supplies, screens the patient, and dons her gloves. She wipes the patient's genitals from front to back with a cotton swab or moist washcloth and cleans the anal regions with a different swab or washcloth. This should be done on each labia at least thrice, and then the labia should be carefully dried. CNAs should be observant of any signs of discomfort or pain during perineal care. Any signs of pain or discomfort should be reported to a nurse or physician for further evaluation.

- **For male patients**

All principles of handwashing and privacy should be followed first, and then the CNA should wipe the genital area and observe for circumcision status to determine how to clean the foreskin to prevent infection. The focus should be on ensuring the area is cleaned effectively and hygienically. The number of times and the method used can vary depending on the individual patient's needs and the resources available. The primary goal is to maintain cleanliness and prevent infection while respecting the patient's comfort and dignity.

Catheter care is another vital part of perineal care. It is to be done daily and requires patient education, consent, and privacy.

Clients should be well positioned and made comfortable. Drainage bags should be emptied, and patients should not be too exposed. This means that only the site to be cleaned should be uncovered. The CNA should use a washcloth and a mild soap to clean the urethral region. Afterward, the catheter should be cleaned with downward strokes and then gently wiped with another cloth.

Abnormalities should be observed and reported. All procedures must be documented.

<u>Foot or Nail Care</u>

Foot or nail care is important for patients, especially those with peripheral vascular disease. It helps to keep the feet and nails clean and dry, stimulate adequate blood circulation to the feet, and inspect the skin for signs of pressure or breakage.

Procedures for foot care

The CNA needs to gather a nail file, basin of water (room temperature), soap, lotion, towels, footpowder, and socks (if needed). The patient is prepared for the procedure, consent is obtained, and the feet are then soaked in a basin of warm water.

Next, the CNA washes the skin with soap and massages the areas between the toes while the nails are cleaned. This ensures that bacteria are removed and that circulation is stimulated. The feet are rinsed in another bowl of clean water and dried with a clean towel. CNAs should exercise caution when trimming or filing nails, especially for patients with diabetes or peripheral vascular disease, as they are at higher risk for foot complications. In many healthcare settings, CNAs are not permitted to trim the nails of these patients due to the risk of causing cuts or infections. Nail care in such patients is usually managed by a healthcare professional with specialized training, such as a podiatrist. CNAs can clean the nails and apply moisturizer but should refer to a nurse or podiatrist for nail trimming and filing when necessary. Foot powder can then be applied.

Mouth Care

Mouth care is a hygienic procedure that keeps the teeth in good condition, clears the oral cavity of debris, prevents mouth odors, and moistens dry mouths. Consistent mouth care also facilitates rapid healing after mouth surgery and prevents cracked lips. Patients are encouraged to participate in the procedure.

To care for the mouth, a towel, bowl, disposable gloves, oral spatula, mouth gag, tongue depressor, cotton swab, toothbrush, warm water, denture cleaner, and cotton balls are used. Patients who cannot sit upright are positioned on their side for easy drainage of water from the mouth. Next, a CNA should put on gloves, seek consent, and explain the procedure to the client. Then, a cloth is placed under the chin to avoid soiling clothes.

For patients who are conscious and alert, mouthwash is handed to them in a cup to rinse out the mouth after the procedure. The CNA places a pea-sized amount of toothpaste on a toothbrush and either brushes all surfaces of teeth or assists patients in doing so. They instruct the patient to rinse their mouth and spit in an emesis bowl twice while the gums and mouth are thoroughly cleaned. Then the mouth is wiped with a swab, and the lips are cleaned and moisturized.

When cleaning a patient's dentures, CNAs should use a denture cleaner rather than toothpaste or mouthwash. Toothpaste can be abrasive and may damage the surface of dentures. Mouthwash is not designed for cleaning dentures and may not effectively remove debris or bacteria. After cleaning, dentures should be rinsed thoroughly before being reinserted into the patient's mouth. The dentures must be carefully handled to prevent damage and bacterial infections.

Skin Care

Skin care goes beyond procedures such as baths. It extends to hydration, which involves adequate intake of water. Also, it comprises the use of dermatologist-recommended lotions and ointments for patients daily to avoid peeling and cracking of the skin.

CNAs assist patients with daily skin care activities or encourage them to perform the activities independently.

Toileting

CNAs should consider factors that can affect toileting, such as limited mobility, poor coordination, and degenerative diseases.

It is necessary to support patients with the toileting process, make them feel loved as much as possible, provide comfort, and ensure safety and proper hygiene. Patients who can access the toilet alone should be monitored by a CNA, with assistive toilet devices or emergency signals in place.

CNAs should ensure that toilets are easily accessible and cleaned thoroughly with disinfectants. After every toilet visit, CNAs should clean up or instruct patients to do so under supervision. Some patients might require the use of bedpans. CNAs must have the required skills to help the patient to use bedpans as needed. Catheters, adult diapers, or pads are used to manage incontinence.

CNAs also observe bowel movements to ascertain whether there is a need for dietary changes or further medical care.

Grooming

CNAs can assist with basic grooming tasks like hair washing. CNAs can support the patient's personal grooming preferences within their professional boundaries and based on the individualized needs of the patient.

Dressing or Undressing

Dressing and undressing involve communication between CNAs and patients to ensure that they are comfortable and clothes are not too tight or loose.

Proper positioning of a patient is done before dressing and undressing. This involves consent and the provision of privacy. CNAs turn patients from side to side and gently dress them while taking note of any discomfort or pain.

Patients who can independently dress themselves are only monitored. They can choose what to wear but should be guided if it is not appropriate due to weather conditions. Cultural beliefs should be acknowledged by CNAs since some individuals wear clothes relevant to their traditions.

Patients who require ambulatory care and assistance with dressing may need support in maintaining balance or standing safely. For dressing assistance, CNAs might help patients to sit on a chair or at the edge of the bed and provide support as needed based on the patient's mobility and balance. They may also need encouragement.

Health Maintenance or Restoration

Promote Circulation and Skin Integrity

The integumentary system works directly with the circulatory system because certain substances can enter the bloodstream through capillary networks. When there is a break in the skin, the circulatory system can be impacted. This affects wound healing and determines how long restoration of the integumentary system will take.

Nurses develop care plans to prevent pressure sores, provide comfort, and collaborate with other healthcare providers. For cases of pressure sores, the wound-healing process is influenced by age, nutritional deficiencies, skin integrity, and hypoxia, among other things. CNAs assist nurses with the execution of these plans.

Unconscious patients or patients immobilized due to stroke, paralysis, general body weakness, anemia, amputation, etc., are at risk of skin breakdown and pressure sores.

CNAs must:

- Ensure proper positioning based on the patient's condition, either hourly or daily. This assists circulation and musculoskeletal balance. It also prevents complications and pain.
- Provide air or water mattresses to ensure that pressure will be distributed equally in all directions.
- Respond to different patients' skin care needs.
- CNAs may assist with the use of diapers and catheters, but it's important to note that improper or prolonged use of these can actually negatively impact skin health. The use of diapers and catheters requires careful monitoring to prevent skin irritation, breakdown, and infection. The goal is to manage incontinence while also ensuring that the skin remains clean, dry, and intact.
- Monitor the skin for redness, discoloration, and sores, especially in areas prone to sores (e.g., ischial tuberosities, back of the head, elbows, shoulders, ankles, heels, vertebral spine, etc.).
- Regularly change soiled bedsheets, linens, catheters, etc.
- CNAs may assist with the application of basic skin care products. They should follow the care plan and instructions provided by the nursing staff and report any skin issues they observe.

- Provide comfort to patients with devices such as rubber air rings, cotton rings, fracture boards, wheelchairs, etc.

Nutrition and Hydration

- **Basic nutritional and hydration needs**

Basic nutritional and hydration needs for patients are important to sustain total well-being. A meal plan is prepared based on the unique needs of each patient.

CNAs observe and report on patients' health needs, including dietary needs. CNAs can assist in implementing the prescribed dietary plans and monitoring the patient's response to these plans. For example, a patient who has been diagnosed with diabetes mellitus will have a carbohydrate-restricted meal plan.

Diet is planned with considerations for age, sex, and medical needs. Meals must be provided to patients at the right time and monitored as appropriate.

Patients are allowed to select their food preferences to make them feel welcomed and participate in their care. CNAs must ensure that clean, fresh water is provided with every meal.

Signs of malnutrition and dehydration (e.g., dark urine, dry mouth, constipation, dry skin, etc.) should be monitored by the CNA and reported to the physician. CNAs can measure daily fluid intake and ensure that patients drink the required amount.

Specific dietary health education can also be included in the routine.

- **Factors that affect dietary preferences**

Dietary preferences can be influenced by various factors, including culture and religion.

Religions may have dietary regulations, such as restrictions for the consumption of beef, pork, blooded animals, snails, etc. Consumption of certain plants is also restricted based on religious beliefs and practices among different people.

Other factors that affect dietary intake include:

- Personal choice.
- Allergies and medical conditions.
- Socioeconomic status.

- Environmental influences.
- Awareness of various diets and their benefits.
- Food advertisements, availability, and market trends.

CNAs must note these factors, which can vary from person to person, and adapt specialized care based on an individual's dietary preferences.

- **Factors that affect dietary intake**

As people age, their nutritional needs change, and this affects their choice of food. Health conditions associated with old age, like diabetes, heart disease, eye disorders, or food allergies, can demand specific dietary restrictions.

Also, certain medications can affect appetite, taste perception, or nutrient absorption, thereby influencing dietary intake.

The condition of the mouth, including dental problems or discomfort, can influence a person's ability to chew and enjoy certain foods, which could impact dietary preferences. For example, individuals with gingivitis, loss of teeth, infections of the oral cavity, etc., may struggle to eat hard foods. Also, difficulty in swallowing, known as dysphagia, can restrict food options and require modifications to the texture and consistency of foods. Certain foods have to be boiled extra soft, crushed, or given in liquid form to encourage proper nutrition.

- **Specialized nutrition and hydration care**

Therapeutic diets are carefully crafted meal regimens made to address specific health issues, such as diabetes, heart disease, or renal issues. To provide patients with the proper balance of nutrients to effectively treat their disease, these diets place a strong emphasis on regulating nutrient intake.

For patients with dysphagia, altered-consistency meals are an important component of specialized nutrition and hydration treatment. These plans alter the consistency and viscosity of foods and beverages to make them easier to swallow and lower the risk of choking and aspiration pneumonia.

Healthcare experts, such as dietitians, speech-language pathologists, and doctors, must work closely together to plan therapeutic diets and altered-consistency meals. To create individualized nutrition and hydration programs, these experts consider a patient's particular requirements, tastes, and medical background.

Sleep and Rest Needs

Good sleep and rest enhance brain function, mental health, and fitness. CNAs have a supportive role in executing the care plans for the patient's sleep and rest needs. They help ensure the environment is conducive to sleep, assist with bedtime routines, and observe and report any issues related to sleep.

Issues such as noise, heat, cold, uncomfortable mattresses, etc., should be addressed. Some patients may need specialized equipment, such as cradles, sandbags, etc.

Patients may suffer from sleep disorders or disturbances, such as insomnia or sleep apnea, so CNAs should recognize these problems and collaborate with other healthcare experts to create effective treatment strategies. CNAs are not qualified to recommend or administer medications for sleep disorders or disturbances. The decision to use medication for sleep-related issues is made by physicians or other licensed healthcare providers. While CNAs can assist with non-pharmacological interventions such as creating a restful environment or helping with relaxation techniques, they do not have the authority to suggest or implement therapeutic massages unless specifically trained and authorized to do so within their scope of practice. Any therapeutic interventions for sleep issues should be directed by and carried out under the supervision of qualified healthcare professionals.

Additionally, daily naps are important, particularly for individuals who might not receive enough sleep at night.

Elimination

The elimination of waste materials from the body occurs through the bowels and the bladder. CNAs are expected to have a fundamental knowledge of these processes to provide quality care in the management of patients.

- **Normal elimination patterns**

Bowel movements are influenced by factors that include underlying health problems such as diarrhea, dysentery, constipation, etc. Stool is expected to be brown, formed, and regular. However, bowel movements vary among individuals for different reasons.

The consistency of feces is dependent on diet, bowel functions or disorders, etc.

When the bladder is full, the brain sends signals to the muscles that regulate the bladder, and the person then feels the need to urinate. The frequency of urination in adults can vary widely and is influenced by many factors including fluid intake, bladder capacity, and individual differences. It is common for adults to urinate around six to eight times in a 24-hour period. The typical bladder capacity is about 400 to 600 ml, and the urge to void often occurs well before reaching maximum capacity.

Frequent urination and difficulty with urine control may indicate impairment of renal functions, urinary incontinence or polyuria, proteinuria, hematuria, etc.

- **Promote elimination**

To promote elimination, CNAs must educate patients on the appropriate health behaviors associated with elimination patterns. These habits are centered on:

  - Consumption of a fiber-rich diet, such as fruits, vegetables, and whole grains (wheat, sorghum, etc.). This aids digestion, prevents constipation, and makes stools soft and easy to pass through the anus without hemorrhoids.
  - Consumption of lots of water and fluids to aid bowel movements and micturition. The recommended daily water intake can vary depending on several factors including age, gender, climate, physical activity level, and overall health. Eight 8-ounce glasses of water a day (about 1.9 liters) is a common general guideline. The U.S. National Academies of Sciences, Engineering, and Medicine suggest a total daily water intake of about 3.7 liters (about 15.5 cups) for men and 2.7 liters (about 11.5 cups) for women, which includes all beverages and water-rich foods.
  - Avoidance of harmful practices like delayed defecation or urination. This habit can lead to chronic constipation and damage the pelvic floor muscles.
  - Physical exercises that should be included in the activities of patients to aid bowel and bladder movements.
  - Lessened consumption of alcohol and caffeine, which can impact bladder function.

- **Bowel and bladder training principles**

Bowel and bladder training are strategies used to regain control over these body functions, especially in cases of incontinence or abnormal elimination patterns.

The nurse is expected to establish the following principles, and CNAs should assist patients to adapt to these changes.

- For bowel and bladder training, CNAs should set a time for bowel and bladder movements depending on patient needs, preferably after meals. This will help to train the bladder to hold urine for longer periods.
- CNAs can assist with non-invasive bowel and bladder training techniques and support the overall care plan. They also help with the use of suppositories, enemas, or laxatives, as directed by the supervisor.
- Encourage fluid and fiber intake in between meals to aid digestion.
- Encourage patients to participate in exercises and relaxation therapies, such as bladder training, to improve muscle control.
- Monitor urine and bowel movement patterns, record volumes, and report abnormalities to the healthcare providers.

Mobility

- **Promote mobility and proper positioning.**

Good mobility and proper positioning are vital to ensure the overall well-being and quality of life of patients in nursing homes and care facilities. This approach incorporates a range of techniques and devices.

- **Importance of mobility and proper positioning.**

For patients in healthcare facilities, particularly those with physical disabilities, chronic illnesses, or in recovery from surgery, bed mobility, and correct positioning are vital for several reasons:

- Prevent complications: Immobility can lead to complications, including pressure ulcers and muscle atrophy, and joint contractures and proper positioning help eliminate or reduce these risks.
- Enhance quality of life: When patients can move freely and comfortably, they can participate in daily activities. This promotes independence to perform self-care activities related to hygiene, feeding, and toileting.
- Improve mental health: When patients can change positions and move around, it can positively impact their mental health. It reduces feelings of helplessness and boosts their overall mood and self-esteem.

The role of CNAs

CNAs help with the promotion of mobility and proper positioning among patients. They must collaborate with physical therapists, occupational therapists, and aides. Here are some major responsibilities of CNAs:

- **Assess**: CNAs assist in observing and reporting on patients' mobility levels, physical limitations, and positioning needs. This assessment, which is made from the client's history, forms the basis for personal care plans.
- **Plan and Implement**: Based on assessments, care plans are created to address patients' specific needs. These plans include strategies for mobility exercises, repositioning schedules, and the use of assistive and comfort devices. CNAs assist in the implementation of care plans that are developed by healthcare professionals. They follow the established care plans, provide direct patient care, and communicate any observations or concerns to the nursing staff or therapists who are responsible for adjusting the care plan as needed.
- **Educate**: CNAs educate both patients and their caregivers about the importance of mobility and proper positioning. They also teach patients techniques to enhance their mobility, report abnormalities, and ensure correct positioning at all times.
- **Monitor and Adjust**: It is essential to monitor patients' mobility and positioning regularly. CNAs assess the effectiveness of interventions and make necessary recommendations to the nurses on the care plans.

Common positions include:

- Left lateral position.
- Prone position.
- Semi-prone position.
- Recumbent or dorsal position.
- Semi-recumbent position.
- Semi-fowler's position.
- Sim's position.
- Supine position.
- Lithotomy position.
- Genu-pectoral position.
- Trendelenburg's position.

- **Promote mobility.**

Healthcare facilities utilize a range of interventions and devices, including prosthetic and orthotic devices. For patients with limb amputations or musculoskeletal issues, prosthetic and orthotic devices enhance mobility and provide proper support.

- **Ensure safe transfer techniques.**

CNAs are trained in safe transfer techniques, which involve assisting patients to safely move from one surface to another, such as from a bed to a wheelchair, stretcher, etc.

This can be achieved with:

  - Electric patient lifts.
  - Manual patient lifts, wherein the CNA must:
    - CNAs are trained in assisting with patient transfers using manual patient lifts. Safe transfer techniques include the use of equipment like a Hoyer lift or a gait belt, and the focus is on assisting the patient rather than lifting them entirely. The goal is to ensure the safety of both the patient and the caregiver, and to avoid injury or strain.
    - Turn a patient on their side.
    - Move a patient from one side of the bed to another.
    - Lift the injured extremity carefully and gently.

- **Use devices that promote mobility.**

Devices like braces, walkers, wheelchairs, and gait belts are employed to assist patients with mobility. These aids are selected based on individual needs and abilities to assist with movement and promote participation in daily life activities.

Trapeze bars installed over beds help patients to reposition themselves comfortably, which reduces the need for continuous assistance.

- **Range-of-motion techniques.**

CNAs may assist in range-of-motion exercises as directed by physical therapists or nurses. These exercises are unique to patients' needs. For instance, someone with impairment of the lower limbs will not perform the same exercise as someone with upper limb discomfort.

Effects of Immobility

- **Impaired circulation and skin integrity.**

Immobility can lead to reduced blood circulation, which increases the risk of pressure ulcers. CNAs check for sores, bleeding, redness, and edema and then establish individualized care.

- **Impaired elimination.**

Immobility can result in constipation and urinary retention. CNAs encourage a balanced diet, ensure regular toileting schedules, and monitor for signs of urinary tract infections.

- **Impaired sleep and rest patterns.**

CNAs create a comfortable sleep environment, promote relaxation techniques, and assess for pain or discomfort, which might impact sleep.

- **Lowered self-image.**

Patients who have just had a change of lifestyle, physical changes, and changes in psychosocial relationships might experience low self-esteem and disturbed self-image. For example, a previously active man who becomes idle due to old age is likely to suffer emotional distress.

CNAs provide emotional support, encourage self-care activities, and involve patients in decision-making about their care.

- **Lessened strength and endurance.**

Immobility can cause muscle atrophy and decreased strength. CNAs work with nurses and physiotherapists to ensure the execution of individualized exercise programs to maintain muscle strength and mobility.

- **Reduced activity tolerance.**

Due to immobility, a person's participation in activities may be reduced. For example, an amputee will gradually be trained on how to use a wheelchair, crutches, communication devices, etc. CNAs develop strategies to gradually increase activity levels, encourage mobility as tolerated, and monitor vital signs, especially pulse and blood pressure, during activities.

- **Lessened comfort.**

When one is unable to move and is fixed to a position, it can lead to discomfort and pain. There is a likelihood of pressure sores, joint aches, etc. CNAs can observe and report on the patient's pain levels and comfort.

Care and Use of Assistive Devices

Many patients rely on assistive devices to maintain their independence and enhance their quality of life.

These devices are:

- **Mobility devices**: Patients are provided with devices such as wheelchairs, crutches, and rods to assist them with movement. CNAs should observe and report any issues with mobility devices such as wheelchairs and crutches. Patients should be educated on how to use and care for these devices.
- **Audio/Visual aids**: Audio aids are used to assist patients with hearing and visual disabilities. Hearing aids, magnifiers, eyeglasses, etc., are examples of aids. CNAs may assist in cleaning audio/visual aids and ensuring they are in good working order. Furthermore, they can remind patients or nursing staff when batteries need replacement and assist in facilitating this process. Patients should be educated on how to use the devices and protect them from damage.
- **Bathroom assistive devices**: Grab railings, raised toilet seats, bathroom mats, and shower chairs help patients with mobility impairment maintain their hygiene independently. CNAs should inspect these devices regularly to ensure they are properly installed and in good condition. They should ensure that they assist patients to use these devices suitably.
- **Feeding aids**: For patients with difficulty swallowing or medical conditions that impede grip, adaptive feeding aids like special utensils, plates, and cups are essential. CNAs should monitor the care of these feeding aids before and after use. Also, patients should be taught how to make use of these devices so that they can feed independently.
- **Devices adapted to promote self-care**: Patients with cognitive impairments may benefit from memory aids like medication reminders, calendars, or visual schedules.
- **Devices for comfort**: Patients make use of devices for comfort, such as special cushions, sandbags, air rings, pillows, bed rails, trapeze, etc. For

example, patients who spend a considerable amount of time in bed or in chairs need these devices to enhance their comfort and prevent pressure sores. These assistive devices should be regularly cleaned, replaced when worn, and adapted to meet individual comfort needs.

Chapter 4: Basic Nursing Care

CNAs should understand basic nursing care practices so they can render care to patients as needed.

Routine, Chronic, Non-life-threatening Situations

Observe and Report Physical Changes

CNAs are expected to observe and report physical changes in patients, so knowledge of anatomy and physiology is essential.

Basic anatomy and functions of the body systems

The human body is composed of various organs, tissues, and cells, which can be categorized into several body systems, each with unique functions and contributions to overall health. These systems include:

1. The musculoskeletal system (muscles, bones and joints)

The body contains 206 bones, and they are further classified according to shape: the long bones (femur, humerus, radius), short bones (tarsals, carpals), flat bones (ribs, sternum), and irregular bones (mandible, vertebrae, ear ossicles).

Bones consist of articulations known as joints.

The skeletal system provides structural support and protection for vital organs and facilitates movement. It is made of bones, joints, and cartilage. The skeleton is divided into two parts:

Axial skeleton: This forms the longitudinal axis of the body, the skull, the vertebral column, and the bony thorax.

Appendicular skeleton: This is composed of 126 bones of the limbs and the pectoral and pelvic girdles, which attach to the limbs of the axial skeleton.

Bones store minerals, produce blood cells, and support the body's weight, while joints enable mobility. Muscles are also responsible for movement. There are three types of muscles: skeletal (voluntary), smooth (involuntary), and cardiac (heart). Muscles also help maintain body posture and generate heat.

The joints are classified into:

Fibrous joints: These joints are fixed, e.g., skull sutures.

Cartilaginous joints: These are slightly movable joints, such as the vertebral joints.

Synovial joints: Synovial joints, or diarthroses, are freely movable joints, but they are not exclusively found in the mandible, shoulders, and knees. Synovial joints are present in many parts of the body, including the hips, elbows, wrists, and ankles. These joints are characterized by a synovial cavity filled with fluid, which allows for a wide range of motion.

Common disorders and conditions that affect the musculoskeletal system

Some common disorders and conditions that affect the musculoskeletal system include:

Rheumatoid arthritis: This is a chronic inflammatory or autoimmune disease that affects the joints. In this condition, the immune system attacks the synovial joints, which leads to inflammation, thickening, and accumulation of fluid in the joint space. The accumulation of these substances in the joint forms scarred, fibrous tissue, and this erodes the cartilage and destroys the joint, which causes stiffness and pain. Rheumatoid arthritis is characterized by painful joints, fatigue, decrease in range of motion, swelling, and smooth and shiny skin of the affected joints.

Roles of CNAs in the management of rheumatoid arthritis

CNAs are expected to be familiar with the disease process and encourage patients to rest. They must also provide all physician-ordered measures to control pain and fatigue. CNAs assist patients with movement and exercises to increase circulation and relieve pain. This also applies to the immobilization of acutely inflamed joints.

Osteoporosis: Osteoporosis is a disorder of bone metabolism that leads to a reduction in total bone mass. It is common in the elderly and affects bone formation, which leaves the bones brittle and weak. The affected bones lose calcium and phosphate salts, and they become porous and prone to fractures. Osteoporosis is primarily caused by a decrease in bone density and strength, which can be due to factors such as aging, hormonal changes (especially in postmenopausal women), genetic predisposition, and dietary deficiencies (particularly calcium and vitamin D). Prolonged immobilization and malnutrition can contribute to the loss of bone density. Additionally, certain liver conditions can be associated with bone loss. Rheumatoid arthritis is a risk factor for secondary osteoporosis due to inflammation and the use of certain medications like corticosteroids.

Roles of CNAs in the management of osteoporosis

CNAs must adhere to safety precautions in the management of patients with osteoporosis. Bedrails should be fixed, and affected bones must be handled with great care to prevent fractures.

Also, CNAs assist patients with measures to aid bowel and bladder elimination since they are prone to constipation and paralytic ileus. Wound dressing is important if there are any breaks in the skin, and hourly client positioning should be done to prevent pressure sores.

Fractures: Fractures are traumatic musculoskeletal injuries that lead to an interruption of bone continuity. They are caused by bone weakness, extreme bone crushing due to accidents, and prolonged bed rest or muscle disuse. When undue stress is placed on a bone, this leads to injury to the blood vessels, periosteum, and surrounding tissues, which then causes bleeding and inflammation of the affected area.

Roles of CNAs in the management of fractures

CNAs provide care and assist in the rehabilitation of clients with fractures. They evaluate and report pain intensity, monitor vital signs, and observe any difficulty in breathing due to pain. Patients with fractures should have their mobility observed from time to time, and self-care practices, such as oral and body hygiene, should be promoted.

Amputation: Amputation is the total or partial surgical removal of a part of the body, such as the upper or lower extremities, digits, or limbs. Amputation may occur as a result of a malignant tumor, inadequate tissue perfusion, trauma, peripheral vascular disease, etc.

Roles of CNAs in the management of amputation

Mobility assistance, emotional support, and observation of vital signs are key roles of the CNA in the management of amputation. CNAs assist with activities of daily living and dress wounds appropriately to prevent infection. They also help patients to put on and remove prosthetic devices.

Dislocation: This is the displacement of a bone from its normal articulation with a joint. Common sites of dislocation include the shoulder, elbow, wrist, digits, hip, knee, ankle, and vertebra. It can be caused by trauma, congenital displacement, and diseases of the joint. Dislocations can be characterized by extreme pain, edema, disruption of joint function, and impaired joint mobility.

Roles of CNAs in the management of dislocation

CNAs are not usually authorized or trained to immobilize joints or apply bandages, casts, splints, or similar devices for dislocations. CNAs can assist in providing comfort and support to the patient, monitor and report changes in the patient's condition, and follow the care plan as directed by a licensed healthcare professional.

2. The circulatory system (heart and blood vessels)

The circulatory system transports oxygen, nutrients, hormones, and waste products throughout the body. The heart pumps blood through the arteries, veins, and capillaries, which ensures a continuous flow to cells and tissues.

The blood consists of elements suspended in a liquid component (plasma). This plasma constitutes 55% of blood volume and contains large quantities of organic and inorganic substances. In an adult, the total blood volume is approximately 7-8% of the body weight, but this statement about the bone marrow is incorrect. The percentage provided (4 to 5%) is not a measure of the bone marrow's contribution to blood volume. Bone marrow is responsible for producing blood cells, but it does not constitute a percentage of the blood volume. The role of bone marrow is to generate new blood cells, including erythrocytes (red blood cells), leukocytes (white blood cells), and thrombocytes (platelets). The blood cells are made of erythrocytes, leukocytes, and thrombocytes. The immune system is made up of white blood cells, and the lymphatic system defends the body against infections and diseases. White blood cells identify and destroy pathogens, and the lymphatic system transports immune cells and fluids.

The heart is a hollow, muscular organ that lies in the mediastinum and rests on the diaphragm. It is encased in the pericardium, which has spaces that contain fluid between its layers to protect the heart from trauma and friction. The walls of the heart consist of three tissue layers:

Epicardium: The thin, serous outer layer.

Myocardium: The thick, muscular middle layer.

Endocardium: The smooth inner layer that comes in contact with blood.

The heart is made up of two major chambers: the atrium and the ventricle. Through these chambers, blood flows in and out of the heart, and the right atrium receives systemic venous blood through the superior vena cava, inferior vena cava, and coronary sinus. The left atrium receives oxygenated blood back to the heart from the lungs through the pulmonary veins.

The heart also consists of cardiac cells that initiate electrical impulses. The sinoatrial (SA) node functions as a pacemaker for the myocardium and initiates rhythmic electrical impulses. The AV node receives this impulse from the SA node and relays it to the ventricles. This electrical impulse, which moves through the cardiac conduction system, is measured by electrocardiography.

Common disorders of the circulatory system

Peripheral artery disease (PAD): This occurs as a result of the occlusion of arteries, especially in the lower extremities, which may be acute or chronic. It is caused by trauma, embolism, thrombosis, inflammation, or autoimmune response.

Myocardial infarction: This is the destruction of the myocardial tissues in the region of the heart due to a severe deprivation of blood flow and oxygen supply. This could be caused by embolism, hypoxia, hypertension, anemia, or other coronary artery diseases.

The elderly are usually predisposed to myocardial infarction, as are individuals who suffer from diseases such as diabetes mellitus, obesity, excessive stress, etc.

CNAs assist with diagnostic tests and nursing care and also monitor patients' intake.

3. The respiratory system

The respiratory system facilitates the exchange of oxygen (O_2) and carbon dioxide (Co_2). The lungs inhale oxygen and exhale carbon dioxide, which is essential for cellular respiration. Other organs of the respiratory system include the nose, sinuses, pharynx, epiglottis, larynx, trachea, bronchi, and alveolar cells.

Major functions of the respiratory system

The respiratory system is responsible for air conduction to the lower respiratory tract, protection of the lungs, diffusion of gases, pulmonary blood supply, and neurological control.

Common disorders of the respiratory system

Pneumonia: This is an inflammatory process that involves the respiratory bronchioles, alveolar spaces, and lungs. It impairs gas exchange and could lead to little oxygen in the blood. Pneumonia is often caused by bacteria, viral infections, immunosuppression, immobility, aspiration, etc. These infectious organisms trigger the inflammation of the airways, which results in edema, fever, pleuritic chest pain, dyspnea, tachycardia, malaise, etc.

Asthma: This is a reactive airway disorder that leads to airway obstruction and inflammation, bronchospasm, and increased mucous secretion.

For patients with asthmatic conditions, CNAs provide relaxation techniques, monitor the use of inhalers, encourage deep breathing, and assist with oxygen administration.

4. The gastrointestinal system (stomach, intestines, and organs)

The gastrointestinal system consists of the oral structures, stomach, small intestine, large intestine, and associated structures. The oral structures include the lips, teeth, gingival and oral mucosa, tongue, hard and soft palate, pharynx, and salivary glands. The esophagus is a muscular tube that extends from the pharynx to the stomach. The esophagus has two sphincters: the upper esophageal sphincter at its beginning (where it connects to the pharynx) and the lower esophageal sphincter at its end (where it connects to the stomach). These sphincters function to regulate the passage of food and prevent backflow.

The stomach is a muscular pouch situated in the upper abdomen under the liver and the diaphragm. The stomach consists of three anatomic areas, namely the fundus, the body, and the pylorus. The pyloric sphincter regulates the flow of the stomach contents into the duodenum.

The small intestine consists of the duodenum, the jejunum, and the ileum. It is a coiled tube that extends from the pyloric sphincter to the ileocecal valves at the large intestine. The large intestine is a shorter and wider tube, which begins at the ileocecal valve and ends at the anus. The large intestine includes more than just the cecum and the rectum. It begins with the cecum, is followed by the ascending, transverse, descending, and sigmoid colon, and ends with the rectum and anal canal. The large intestine is responsible for absorbing water and electrolytes from undigested food material and for the formation and elimination of feces.

Functions of the gastrointestinal system

The GI system processes food and extracts nutrients and energy before waste is eliminated. Organs like the stomach, liver, and pancreas aid in digestion and nutrient absorption.

Common disorders of the gastrointestinal system

Peptic ulcer: Peptic ulcers are sores that develop on the lining of the stomach, lower esophagus, or small intestine. They occur in the stomach and the duodenum (the first part of the small intestine). The term "pylorus" refers to the pyloric region of the stomach, but it's more precise to mention the stomach and duodenum separately when discussing peptic ulcers. The ulcers are commonly caused by an infection with Helicobacter pylori bacteria and long-term use of NSAIDs (nonsteroidal anti-inflammatory drugs). They are caused by bacteria, certain drugs such as NSAIDs, alcohol ingestion, stress, and genetic predisposition. CNAs monitor the feeding patterns of patients with peptic ulcers and encourage rest.

CNAs should also assist with patient feeding if necessary, monitor bowel movements, provide routine vital sign checks, as well as clean out feeding tubes and dress wounds as necessary.

Malnutrition: Malnutrition is a common indication of gastrointestinal disorders. It leads to fluid volume deficit, impaired skin integrity, and disturbed body image.

For cases associated with feeding disorders in patients with gastrointestinal disorders, enteral tubes are used to administer feedings, fluids, and medications. These tubes are made for gastric decompression and drainage and also to lessen patient discomfort and nasal irritation.

The frequency of replacing enteral tubes depends on the type of tube, the patient's condition, and the healthcare facility's protocols. Some enteral tubes may need to be replaced periodically, while others are designed for longer-term use. CNAs ensure that whatever fluid or formula is introduced into the GIT meets the nutritional needs of the patient.

5. The nervous system (brain, spinal cord, and nerves)

The central nervous system is made up of protective cranial structures. The brain is enclosed by the bones of the cranium and covered by three meningeal layers: the dura mater, arachnoid mater, and pia mater. The cerebrospinal fluid circulates in the subarachnoid space and is manufactured in the choroid plexus of the ventricular system.

The brain is divided into distinct areas: the cerebrum, cerebellum, and brainstem (composed of the midbrain, pons, and medulla oblongata). The lobes contained within each left and right cerebral hemisphere are described as frontal, temporal, parietal, and occipital. The cerebellum is divided into left and right hemispheres and connected by the vermis. It is located beneath the cerebral hemispheres and separated from them by a structure known as the tentorium cerebelli, which is an extension of the dura mater. The tentorium cerebelli is a horizontal fold of dura mater that creates a separation between the cerebrum and the cerebellum.

Functions of the nervous system

The nervous system controls and coordinates body functions. The brain processes information while the spinal cord relays messages between the brain and the rest of the body. This makes up the central nervous system. The peripheral nervous system consists of the cranial and spinal nerves and transmits signals to muscles and organs, which allows for voluntary and involuntary actions.

The brainstem, which includes the midbrain, pons, and medulla oblongata, is located at the base of the brain and is connected to the spinal cord. While it does contain the reticular formation, the brainstem is not solely comprised of this. The reticular formation is a network of neurons within the brainstem that regulates wakefulness and sleep-wake transitions. The brainstem as a whole is responsible for many vital functions, including heart rate, breathing, sleeping, and eating. The brain consists of structures that help stabilize cranial structures, determine cognitive function, control sensory organs, and maintain balance (muscle tone and equilibrium). The hypothalamus in the brain also regulates temperature, fluid balance, and some endocrine functions.

Common disorders of the nervous system

Stroke: Stroke is a condition in which neurologic deficit results from decreased blood flow to a localized area of the brain. This causes a reduction in oxygen supply and serious damage and necrosis of brain tissues. Hemorrhagic stroke also occurs when blood vessels break open, which spills blood into the spaces that surround the neurons.

CNAs assist with mobility, observe response and alertness, and educate clients on movement.

Delirium: Delirium is a mental disorder characterized by confusion, loss of alertness, and psychological imbalance in the elderly.

CNAs provide care, monitor vital signs, and report abnormal findings to the registered nurse. They also assist with activities of daily living, hygiene, and bowel and bladder care.

6. The urinary system (kidneys and bladder)

The urinary system consists of the kidneys, ureters, bladder, and urethra. The kidneys filter blood and produce urine, the ureters transport urine from the kidneys to the bladder, the bladder stores urine, and the urethra is the channel through which urine is discharged from the body. The ureters are slender tubes that extend behind the peritoneum from the hilus of the kidney to the bladder. The bladder is a smooth, collapsible muscular sac located in the pelvis and connects to the urethra. The urethra is the tube that leads from the bladder to the outside of the body and allows urine to be excreted. The kidneys are located on either side of the vertebral column, but it should be clarified that they are situated in the posterior part of the abdomen, against the back muscles, and are retroperitoneal (located behind the peritoneum).

External structures of the kidney

The medial border of the kidney is indented by the renal hilum, which is the entry and exit point for the renal artery, renal vein, lymphatic vessels, nerves, and the ureter. The renal hilum leads to a space within the kidney known as the renal sinus, which houses these structures. The kidneys are also made up of a fibrous transparent outer covering called the renal capsule.

Inner structures of the kidney

Cortex: Glomerulus, tubules, and part of Henle's loop.

Medulla: Henle's loop and the collecting ducts.

Renal pyramids: Collecting ducts with bases on the border between the cortex and medulla.

The nephron: A functional unit of the kidney that contains glomeruli, tubules, and collecting ducts.

Functions of the urinary system

The urinary system is responsible for the removal of waste and excess substances from the body through urine formation and transportation to the bladder. Kidneys filter blood and maintain electrolyte balance while the bladder stores and excretes urine. The kidneys are also responsible for the metabolism of vitamin D and regulate red blood cell production by erythropoietin secretion.

Common disorders of the urinary system

Urinary tract infection (UTI): UTIs involve infection along the entire urinary tract, whether the upper urinary tract (pyelonephritis) or lower urinary tract infections (cystitis and urethritis). UTIs are caused by microorganisms such as candida, staphylococci, enterobacter, pseudomonas, etc. When these microorganisms multiply, they cause inflammation, and this leads to fever, dysuria, hematuria, pain, incontinence, urgency, etc.

CNAs monitor bladder output, urine color, and amount. They monitor and report vital signs and encourage patients to drink lots of fluid.

Urinary incontinence: This refers to the inability of the urine sphincter to control the release of urine. It is often caused by inflammation, stress, old age, use of medications (diuretics), stroke, immobility, and bladder lesions. Patients with urinary incontinence often present with uncontrolled micturition, anxiety, pruritus, bedwetting, and depression. CNAs may assist with dietary choices and fluid intake for patients, especially those with urinary incontinence. For individuals with mobility impairments, CNAs assist with access to the bathroom (if possible) and clean up after urination.

Characteristics of bodily functions observable by CNAs

The bodily functions that CNAs can observe include a wide range of vital signs, physical characteristics, and behaviors that offer significant indications about a patient's general health and well-being. These observations include vital signs, height, weight, skin integrity, excretion, circulation, dietary intake, mobility, and alignment.

1. Vital signs

Patient's physical functions can be determined by an assessment of their vital signs. They consist of:

Blood pressure: Blood pressure (BP) is measured with a sphygmomanometer and recorded as the ratio of the systolic (pressure during heartbeats) to the diastolic (pressure between heartbeats) pressure. The detection of hypertension or hypotension is aided by normal BP readings. The heart rate is measured by the pulse rate, which is expressed in beats per minute (BPM). Various cardiac or circulation conditions may be indicated by abnormal pulse rates.

Pulse rate: The pulse rate is an important vital sign. The evaluation of a patient's pulse includes assessing the rate (speed), rhythm (regularity), and strength or quality of the pulse. The pulse can be felt in several locations on the body, including the radial artery (at the wrist) and the pedal artery (on the foot). CNAs are trained to check and report on these aspects of the pulse as part of routine vital sign monitoring.

Respiration rate: The rate of breathing is measured in cycles per minute. Respiratory issues might be indicated by deviations from the normal range.

Body temperature: Oral, ear, or axillary procedures are used to measure body temperature. The temperature readings can be used to detect infection, fever, hyperthermia, or hypothermia.

2. Height and weight

A person's height and weight might provide information about their development and dietary needs. Weight is usually expressed in kilograms or pounds, but height is usually measured in centimeters or inches. Deviations from predicted levels may be a sign of obesity or malnutrition.

3. Skin integrity

The skin is the largest organ in the body, and its state reflects general health.

Skin tone: Pale, jaundiced, or cyanotic skin may indicate problems with circulation.

Skin texture: Dry, cracked, or sweaty skin may be a sign of dehydration, malnutrition, or other ailments.

Skin lesions or ulcers: Sores, wounds, or pressure ulcers need to be attended to right away. Failure to heal may signal the need for urgent attention.

4. Elimination

It's important to pay attention to a patient's bowel and bladder routines.

Bowel and bladder movements: The regularity, consistency, and/or presence of blood or mucus during bowel movements can indicate digestive issues. Also, urine color, smell, and specific gravity can help identify urinary tract problems.

5. Circulation

CNAs must observe blood flow and perfusion in order to evaluate circulation. Capillary refill and peripheral edema could point to heart issues or poor circulation.

6. Nutritional intake

CNAs frequently keep track of a patient's food and liquid consumption. This includes the kind and quantity of food consumed, its nutritional content, and the patient's level of hydration.

7. Mobility

CNAs assess a patient's capacity for movement and participation in daily activities. Any obstacles are documented, and joint movement and muscular strength are evaluated. CNAs record whether patients can move freely or need assistive devices (crutches, wheelchairs, etc.).

8. Alignment

Proper body alignment for bedridden people lessens the chance of pressure ulcers and other skin problems, while good posture generally lowers the risk of musculoskeletal issues.

The general health and rehabilitation of their patients are aided by CNAs' rigorous assessment of vital signs, height, weight, skin integrity, elimination, circulation, food intake, mobility, and alignment. This helps to ensure that any deviations from the norm are immediately addressed.

Observe and Report Behavioral Changes

Patients are assessed based on their body build, psychological status, and changes in behavior.

Individual posture, proper grooming, mobility, and other factors, such as unexplained weight loss or choice of clothing, are also observed. Under the right circumstances, patients are expected to appear neat, stable, and maintain a healthy lifestyle. CNAs should observe and report behavioral changes, including changes in clothing choices.

Clothing choices can be influenced by a variety of factors, including personal preference, cultural background, or comfort, and do not necessarily indicate a health concern. Behavioral observations should focus more on changes that are indicative of a patient's mental or physical health, such as drastic changes in hygiene, mobility, or demeanor.

Mental status changes

State of mind is assessed through the verbal and nonverbal patterns of patients. For instance, is the client energetic, confident, sad, discouraged, or indifferent?

A patient who paces constantly around the ward might indicate potential anxiety, disturbance, outrage, and aggression and is graded based on this level. Relevant data about the client is also gathered during the interview, where all preexisting conditions are discussed and presenting symptoms are investigated.

Confusion is visible when a patient needs signals to answer orders and questions or is not situated to their current circumstance. Sluggish patients can be encouraged to perform a task or engage in daily routines, especially self-care activities.

The mental status of patients is assessed with questions and observation of things like a passive nod, selective mutism, indifference to activities, or cognitive impairment. Mental state is assessed through the client's degree of perception, basic knowledge of numerical computations, speech coherence, and ability to respond appropriately to orders and questions.

Emotional stress and mood status changes

A treatment plan provides patients with an atmosphere where self-expression is possible. Judgment or criticism is absent, and healthcare professionals can build a strong relationship with patients.

The most frequently seen psychological and emotional manipulations associated with acute and severe illness are expressions of guilt, anxiety, anger, and distress.

Assessment of emotional stress and mood status changes

The central qualities of anxiety are evident in physiological changes, including shuddering, trembling voice, or twitching. It can also include social changes such as sleep deprivation, fretfulness, vulnerability, dejection, or hopelessness.

Parasympathetic reactions include the body's rest and digestion response. Parasympathetic responses generally include decreased heart rate, increased gastrointestinal activity (which could potentially include diarrhea), and relaxation of muscles. Hyperpnea and anorexia can result from nervousness, and mental side effects like a lessened ability to focus and trepidation can occur.

Assessment of emotional stress and mood status changes include:

Survey the client for emotional and objective signs and side effects of nervousness. The Face Uneasiness Scale can be utilized to assess the client's tension.

Help the patient to replace negative thoughts with positive ones.

Diaphragmatic breathing can help calm anxious patients, as can meditation.

Memory treatment involves the sharing of biographies, recollections, individual memoirs, and chronicles with others. Memory treatment provides the individual with a healthy identity, regard, and worth.

Journaling gives individuals the chance to record their sentiments and thoughts.

Music can be utilized alone or along with deep breathing, meditation, and directed symbolism to calm patients.

Reality orientation or validation

Reality orientation is a technique that helps individuals in long-term care settings to maintain awareness of their surroundings (especially those with cognitive impairments like dementia). Reality orientation reinforces environmental and personal information, such as the current time, date, and location, to assist patients in maintaining a sense of reality. The use of schedules, clocks, and sensory cues can be part of this approach.

Reality validation helps underscore the time, day, month, year, situation, and climate.

Defense mechanisms

Defense mechanisms are psychological strategies used unconsciously to protect a person from anxiety that arises from unacceptable thoughts or feelings. They are automatic psychological processes that protect individuals from anxiety and the awareness of internal or external dangers or stressors. Defense mechanisms can be both healthy and unhealthy, depending on how they are used and their impact on an individual's functioning.

Projection: Projection happens when patients blame someone else for their disappointments. Projection shields the patient's inner self from harm until the person is prepared to adapt to these disappointments.

Withdrawal: Patients detach and withdraw to avoid the stress until they are ready to cope with it.

Sublimation: Sublimation is a defense mechanism where socially unacceptable impulses or idealizations are transformed into socially acceptable actions or behaviors. An example of sublimation would be a person channeling aggressive energies into something productive like sports or a person with strong feelings of aggression working out intensively at the gym as a way to manage these feelings.

Undoing: A person attempts to 'undo' an unacceptable behavior or thought by engaging in a contrary behavior.

Behavioral correction

Behavioral correct can be achieved by:

- The maintenance of a predictable atmosphere, precise timetables, and schedules.
- The promotion of socialization and relaxation activities.
- Physical exercise.

Acute Emergencies

An acute emergency is a condition that requires prompt or immediate short-term medical intervention, the absence of which could result in severe morbidity or mortality. Below are common acute emergencies CNAs should be aware of and know how to respond to.

Chest Pain

Chest pain is often described as tightness, pressure, or sharp pain, and it is usually due to the presence of underlying heart diseases, e.g., myocardial infarction, coronary artery disease, etc.

Age is one factor that predisposes people to these diseases, although conditions such as increased cholesterol, diabetes, hypertension, and genetic or family history can likely lead to the onset of the diseases. Individuals with chest pain usually complain of worsened pain with pressure and shortness of breath.

The onset of chest pain is caused by a lack of oxygen with pain around the sternum, which often radiates to the shoulders. Pain is felt when a nerve ending is stimulated by noxious stimuli and then results in mechanical, thermal, or chemical stimuli.

Nursing interventions for acute chest pain

- Provide relief for patients.
- Assess pain based on location and intensity.
- Place the patient with the head of the bed elevated 45 degrees.
- Administer oxygen as prescribed.
- Monitor vital signs.
- Monitor pain intensity.
- Observe and report indicators of pain such as crying, grimacing, sleeping problems, reduced appetite, and resistance to care.

The roles of CNAs in the management of chest pain

CNAs provide basic care and monitor patients' vital signs and condition. They keep patients comfortable, take vital signs, monitor breathing, and report deviations in vital signs to the nurse or doctor.

Cardiac Arrest

Cardiac arrest is an unexpected termination of the cardiac movements, which leads to unconsciousness, abnormal breathing, and loss of circulation.

Cardiac arrest is mainly caused by cardiovascular diseases, such as ischemic coronary disease, cardiomyopathy, congestive heart failure, dysplasia, etc. It could be a result of respiratory distress, intracranial hemorrhage, sepsis, or traumatic brain injury.

Factors such as obesity, lifestyle (socioeconomic status, occupation, smoking, alcohol dependence), diabetes, family history of cardiovascular diseases, and hypertension are to be documented.

Management of cardiac arrest

The management of cardiac arrest is dependent on the cause. For instance, the management of respiratory distress will most likely require CPR, unlike intracranial hemorrhage, which might require other medical or surgical interventions.

Other nursing management for cardiac arrest includes:

- Assess vitals (temperature, pulse, blood pressure, pulse oximetry) hourly or based on the patient's condition and stability.
- Resuscitate if need be.
- Document all procedures and collaborate with other healthcare providers
- Encourage and assist patients with diagnostic investigations— ECG and blood analysis.
- Insert Foley catheters, especially for unconscious or paralyzed patients.
- Maintain a relaxed atmosphere for patient recovery.

Role of CNAs in the management of cardiac arrest

CNAs take vital signs, observe patients' states, transport immobile patients to the diagnostic laboratory, and assist the nurse with resuscitation and oxygen administration. CNAs should also be skilled in CPR.

Respiratory Distress

Respiratory distress arises when an individual is unable to inhale and exhale air. This is because the body does not receive enough oxygen from the blood, or there is an accumulation of carbon dioxide.

Respiratory distress can occur as a result of obstruction of the upper respiratory tract, in cases of strangulation, drowning, pressure, choking, underlying complications, etc. Also, paralysis of the muscles of respiration in cases of electric shock, poisoning, and inhaled smoke can lead to respiratory distress.

Causes of respiratory distress

Some of the causes of respiratory distress include:

Obstruction of the upper respiratory tract: Blockages of the upper airway can be a result of inflammation, tumors, or foreign materials.

Traumatic incidents: Events such as drowning, fire outbreaks, stampede, strangulation, choking, etc., can all lead to severe respiratory distress.

Presence of underlying disease and infections: Various medical conditions, such as asthmatic attacks, pneumonia, allergic reactions, bronchitis, tuberculosis, chronic obstructive pulmonary disease, lung diseases, etc., can also lead to worsened respiratory distress.

Disorders of the nervous system: Situations that affect the nerves and muscles of coordination can lead to respiratory distress. This includes electric shock and inhalation of gas, carbon monoxide and other toxic chemicals, and poisoning.

Symptoms of respiratory distress

Signs and symptoms of respiratory distress include:

Difficulty breathing: This could include breathlessness, weakness, and forceful breaths.

Also, breathing could be rapid, with evidence of restlessness and a whistling sound in cases of obstructive airway conditions.

Coughing: Individuals with respiratory problems can have chronic coughs, especially when there is an infection of the respiratory tract.

Cyanosis: Cyanosis is characterized by a blue or purplish discoloration of the skin and mucous membranes, due to a lack of oxygen in the blood. The discoloration is most noticeable in areas such as the lips, tongue, and extremities. Individuals with respiratory distress might also have distended veins and dilated pupils. Lack of oxygen can lead to mental confusion and unconsciousness.

Nursing interventions in respiratory distress

CNAs can prepare patients for diagnostic tests such as chest X-rays to reveal abnormalities in the respiratory tract, lung function tests, oxygen saturation measurements, bronchoscopy, and CT scans. These tests help to visualize the airway and detect abnormalities.

Emergency management of respiratory distress

First aid:

- Remove the source of danger, such as a poison or burning object.
- Clear the mouth of obstructions such as blood, vomit, or saliva.
- Artificial respiration and external cardiac massage (CPR) are emergency procedures used to restore normal breathing and circulation. However, the Heimlich maneuver is a specific technique used to dislodge an obstruction from a person's airway when they are choking.

Other management options for respiratory distress

The management of respiratory distress depends on the underlying cause and the severity of the condition. Common treatment options include:

- Oxygen administration as ordered to increase blood oxygen saturation and address cyanosis, mental confusion, and unconsciousness.
- The administration of medications such as antibiotics and bronchodilators.
- Artificial breathing techniques and intubation.
- Collaborate with other healthcare providers in surgical procedures that might involve the removal of respiratory tract obstructions such as tumors.
- Educate patients on the need to identify allergic reactions and prevent the onset of triggers. This includes explanations on the use of inhalers, epinephrine, and face masks.

Role of CNAs in the management of patients with respiratory distress

- CNAs can educate patients on the need for lifestyle changes, such as weight loss or cessation of smoking.
- CNAs monitor vital signs and observe the patient's breathing.
- CNAs remove all the patient's tight clothing, especially around the neck, chest, waist, and abdomen.
- CNAs are expected to conserve the patient's body warmth by placing a blanket underneath and over the individual. This should be monitored so as not to overheat the patient.

Difficulty Swallowing

Dysphagia is a common issue among the elderly. It could be a result of underlying problems such as choking or aspiration.

Often, a change to the texture of a food is implemented. This could be in the form of thickened liquids, mashed food, etc.

Ensure that the patient sits upright when eating and that feeding assistance is given when necessary. As care is ongoing, CNAs are expected to monitor changes in swallowing, hydration, nutritional status, and difficulty in breathing.

CNAs also encourage patients and inform them of the need to report any abnormal sensations.

Choking or Aspiration

Choking obstructs the airway and prevents the flow of air to the lungs. It occurs as a result of stuck food, bones, or foreign substances. A nurse's prompt response is required to clear the airway and restore breathing functions.

Aspiration occurs when foreign substances enter the airway and the lungs. This often leads to lung infections and respiratory problems, e.g., pneumonia.

Nursing interventions for choking or aspiration

- In the case of aspiration, the response depends on the severity and may involve suctioning or medical intervention. Patients should not be laid down in a way that may cause the foreign object to move further into the airway.
- The appropriate first aid response for a choking adult or child is to perform back blows, but these should be done with caution and proper technique. For a conscious person who is choking, the recommended approach is to give 5 back blows followed by 5 abdominal thrusts (Heimlich maneuver), alternating until the blockage is dislodged. This procedure should be performed by someone trained in first aid.
- Seek prompt medical attention and report the situation to the attending physician.
- CPR should be administered in cases of emergency and cessation of breath.
- In cases of respiratory problems from aspiration, oxygen may be administered.
- Monitor vital signs (pulse and respiration) consistently as care continues.

Role of CNAs in the management of choking

CNAs observe breathing patterns, take vital signs, and provide patients with comfort and proper positioning.

Vomiting

Vomiting is a complex reflex involving multiple steps: initially, there is often an increase in salivation, followed by retching (spasmodic respiratory movements against a closed glottis), and finally the expulsion of stomach contents. This process is coordinated by the vomiting center in the brain.

Acute abdominal conditions, fever, gastric disturbances, cerebral conditions that upset the vomiting center in the brain, motion sickness, emotional disturbances, and swallowing of an irritant substance can lead to vomiting.

Vomiting is usually preceded by nausea, cold sweat, increased salivation, gastric pain, and retching. CNAs are required to report characteristics of the vomit that could be life-threatening, such as the presence of blood in the vomit (hematemesis). Also, the odor, color, and manner of expulsion of stomach contents should be noted and reported.

Role of CNAs in the management of vomiting

CNAs assist in positioning the patient when vomiting and provide a clean bowl for vomit. They also measure the amount of vomit, provide assistance with grooming and hygiene, and keep specimens from vomit for laboratory investigations.

Nurses are expected to administer prescribed medications, and CNAs can take vital signs, monitor intake and output, and encourage patients to remain calm throughout the process of care.

Seizures

Seizures are characterized by abnormal, rapid, and uncontrolled neuronal discharges in the brain. Seizures result from excessive electrical activity in the brain, which can affect a person's movements, behavior, feelings, and levels of consciousness.

Seizure disorders, or epilepsy, are not classified solely based on their causes. They are classified by how the seizure manifests (focal or generalized), its origin within the brain, and whether the cause is known or unknown. While brain injury, cerebral edema, hematoma, and raised intracranial pressure can cause seizures, these are specific causes rather than a classification system for seizure disorders. To manage seizure disorders, the nurse identifies the causes and effects, especially factors that predispose an individual to seizures.

Seizures may present as a result of a localized lesion on part of the brain, or they could be generalized and affect the whole body. Often, the nurse addresses the issue of stigma and beliefs about the disorder.

A detailed client history and assessment are done upon admission, which involves childhood or accident history plus other relevant information. Explanations on the importance of medication adherence and follow-up at the clinic are also important.

While it's true that emotional and psychological support is important, it should be noted that there are treatments available for seizure disorders that can effectively manage and, in some cases, completely control seizures. While not all seizure disorders can be cured, many people with epilepsy can lead normal lives with proper medication and treatment.

Role of CNAs in the management of seizures

CNAs can help ensure the safety of a patient experiencing a seizure by removing harmful objects from the vicinity and providing a safe environment. Also, they should observe the general condition of the patient and report to the nurse. This includes the patient's breathing and level of consciousness.

Changes in Mobility, Speech, or Other Potential Signs of Stroke

Changes in mobility, speech, and potential signs of stroke are often neurological disorders that affect the elderly. To assess mobility changes, signs such as weakness, numbness, or loss of coordination are often reported.

Stroke is a condition in which a neurological deficit results from decreased blood flow to a localized area of the brain. This causes a reduction in oxygen supply and serious damage and necrosis of brain tissues.

The FAST (Face, Arms, Speech, Time) test is commonly used to recognize the signs of a stroke: check for facial drooping (Face), arm weakness (Arms), speech difficulties (Speech), and note the time the symptoms started (Time). An inability to lift one or both arms can be a sign of stroke, but it's important to assess all these areas for a comprehensive evaluation.

The nurse carefully observes clinical manifestations, which depend on the affected organ. They could present as paralysis, speech defect, or inability to write or read. Also, urinary incontinence, amnesia, and increased intracranial pressure are major signs of stroke.

CNAs monitor vital signs and assist with bowel and bladder care. CNAs assist with activities of daily living and movement if necessary. They provide bedpans and diapers for patients with urinary incontinence and observe the volume and color of the urine. Abnormalities are reported to the management team.

Nurses monitor intracranial pressure and changes in speech, which are often evidenced by slurred speech or difficulty forming words. A consult with speech and physical therapists is important to begin timely improvement.

Other nursing management for stroke

- Clear the patient's airway and administer oxygen therapy.
- Monitor blood pressure, pulse rate and pulse oximetry, and report and document all abnormalities.
- Assess the patient for neurological function, which may include sensory and motor function.
- Assist as needed with diagnostic imaging tests, such as CT scans and MRIs, to investigate hemorrhage.
- Collaboration with other healthcare providers, such as surgeons, neurologists, dietitians, therapists, etc., is important to provide quality care for patients who have suffered a stroke.
- Ensure fluids and electrolytes are balanced in the body. Monitor hydration (fluid intake and output levels) and perform laboratory investigations (serum electrolyte levels).
- Administer medications, including anticoagulants, or manage intravenous fluids or transfusions. These tasks are performed by licensed nursing staff.
- Educate caregivers on the changes in the patient's status and the need to provide the individual with the necessary support.

Diabetic Situations

Diabetic situations could result in coma due to an excessive increase in the amount of glucose present in the blood (hyperglycemia), breath, and urine. The onset of a diabetic crisis presents with headache, dizziness, restlessness, abdominal pain, deep respiration, and eventual unconsciousness.

The CNA is expected to obtain a detailed history from the client as regards the symptoms of diabetes. This includes the causes, symptoms, past and present medical history, family history, lifestyle, etc. Diabetes can be caused by infections, exposure to drugs and toxins, liver disease, genetic syndromes, excess secretion of hormones (insulin), and dysfunctional insulin receptors in the cells.

In an emergency, a licensed practitioner will administer insulin to diabetic patients. CNAs can assist by recognizing symptoms of hyperglycemia or hypoglycemia and alerting nursing staff or physicians. For circumstances when a patient has not been diagnosed as diabetic, a report is sent to the physician for proper assessment.

Diabetic situations can result in symptoms like confusion, moist skin, and shaky limbs, and these are signs of hypoglycemia (low blood sugar). Fainting and shallow respiration could also be signs of severe hypoglycemia. Often the eventual result of an insulin coma, if not quickly attended to, is unconsciousness. Administration of dextrose intravenous fluids is not a routine treatment for all diabetic situations and should be determined by a healthcare professional. Dextrose is used to treat hypoglycemia. In the case of hyperglycemia, different treatments would be required.

Diabetes parameters to evaluate include:

- Fasting blood glucose: A fasting blood glucose level above 126 mg/dl is generally considered diagnostic of diabetes mellitus, according to the American Diabetes Association. A level of 140 mg/dl after fasting would usually require further testing but is not, on its own, diagnostic of diabetes. Blood glucose levels less than 70 mg/dl are generally considered hypoglycemic and may require attention, especially if symptoms are present. Levels below 60 mg/dl are more concerning and can indicate a need for urgent intervention to prevent severe hypoglycemia.
- Random blood glucose levels.
- Renal function test.
- Urinalysis to reveal glucosuria.
- Serum electrolyte tests, which will reveal hypernatremia and hypokalemia.

The aims of managing diabetes are to maintain blood sugar levels and prevent complications and emergencies associated with the condition. Nutritional management of diabetes includes carbohydrate intake restrictions and a reduction in the intake of refined and simple sugar.

Engaging in activities such as exercise is also important in the management of diabetes, as exercise lowers blood glucose levels and improves insulin sensitivity. Also, monitoring glucose levels is important. The patient is taught how to self-administer insulin and observe glucose level changes, which should be reported accordingly.

Diabetes is a lifelong condition. Therefore, patients and relatives must be educated on how to recognize complications, monitor blood glucose, follow a prescribed diet, and prevent infections as much as possible.

Role of CNAs in the management of diabetic situations

CNAs can help check the patient's blood sugar level and monitor vital signs, but they are not typically authorized to administer insulin. CNAs can assist with other needs and report any changes or concerns to the nursing staff or physicians.

Sudden Onset of Confusion or Agitation

Mental disorders characterized by confusion, loss of alertness, and psychological imbalance are common in the elderly. To manage these conditions, the nurse identifies the causes and presenting symptoms. In the elderly, aged 70 and above, there is a risk of disorders that could lead to confusion, wandering, inability to sleep, anger, and irritability.

CNAs identify the risk of complications or worsening symptoms and report to the nurse. They also assist with personal care and hygiene needs. Hyperactive delirium could be threatening to the individual, relatives, or community. Therefore, relatives are educated on how to manage the situation and follow up on medications.

CNAs provide assistance with activities of daily living, hygiene, and bowel and bladder care. In extreme cases of violence, alterations in vital signs, lack of response to treatment, and fever, CNAs record and report important information and seek to work together with other medical units.

Changes in the Level of Consciousness

Loss of consciousness is when an individual is no longer aware of their surroundings. There are different levels of the unconscious state, such as fully conscious, disoriented to time and space, stupor, coma, etc.

For instance, an individual disoriented to time and space might not know his current location but will be able to answer questions about himself, such as his name and address. In a coma, there is a state of complete unconsciousness, absence of reflexes, and no response to stimuli.

All of these are graded by the nurse, who also identifies the cause of unconsciousness, which could include:

- Anemia.
- Asphyxia.
- Seizure disorders.

- Brain injury and tumors.
- Diabetic coma.
- Cerebrovascular accidents.

CNAs examine patients for hemorrhage, cyanosis, convulsive movements, rapid pulse rates, deep, slow, or shallow, rapid respirations, presence of wounds, odor from the oral cavity, etc. CNAs also observe for discharge from the ears, nose, and bladder.

Generally, the management of changes in the level of consciousness is dependent on the cause. A detailed history of the client is necessary for a thorough assessment. Patients who experience seizures should be placed in a recovery position, which is usually on their side. This position helps keep the airway clear and reduces the risk of aspiration if vomiting occurs.

Likewise, if patients faint, they should be exposed to enough air to allow for circulation, placed in a prone position, and have their mouth suctioned. If unconsciousness is a result of hemorrhage, fracture, or difficulty in breathing, these factors must be addressed and managed appropriately.

CNA interventions for unconscious patients

CNAs position patients to prevent pressure sores, promote circulation, and prevent muscular and joint contractures. They provide bed baths, daily hygiene, and groom patients when necessary.

CNAs may assist with feeding patients orally or with tube feeding. CNAs can also assist with basic oral care. Throat suctioning is a more invasive procedure usually performed by nurses or respiratory therapists. CNAs are expected to clean out catheters regularly and observe and record urine abnormalities. CNAs should report the presence of blood in stool, as it can be a sign of a serious medical condition.

CNAs monitor the vitals and recovery process of each patient. This is to ensure that a thorough reassessment can be made in case of negative outcomes of interventions.

Falls

Functional issues of the musculoskeletal system affect posture, movement of the upper and lower extremities, etc., in all age groups. Falls can also be peculiar to individuals who have certain underlying cardiovascular or neurological disorders.

Gait disorders can be evaluated in elderly patients or individuals who have a history of falls, dementia, stroke, or lack of coordination of nerves and muscles.

The basic movement ability of a person can be impaired after a surgical procedure or when certain traumatic events occur, such as osteoarthritis, chronic diseases, brain injury, etc. This is referred to as immobility, which is a major point of concern for the medical or surgical team and other disciplines within the hospital.

Mobility, which includes movement of the upper and lower limbs and the ability of the patient to adjust in bed and perform various functions, is vital. Therefore, CNAs serve as assistants for patients and encourage exercises that promote mobility.

The first assessment a CNA performs is to observe the patient's posture, mental and physical state, and underlying diseases that can affect movement or cause immobility.

CNAs assist patients to change position in bed from time to time, do active exercises, and monitor improvements in mobility. CNAs can assist with rehabilitation and ambulatory services under the supervision of healthcare professionals. Rehabilitation involves a team of healthcare providers, including physical therapists, occupational therapists, and nurses.

CNAs assess patients with neurological disorders, cardiovascular diseases, and renal impairments for signs and symptoms such as loss of consciousness, hypotension, dizziness, confusion, and lack of mental alertness. They carry out whatever instructions are directed by the nurse and other members of the management team.

Bleeding

Bleeding is an escape of blood from the blood vessels. Hemorrhage could involve internal and external blood vessels. For example, when blood escapes from the blood vessels and can be seen on the skin surface, it is external, while blood that gushes out of the blood vessels into another organ, tissue, or cavity is caused by internal factors.

Hemorrhage is caused by direct injury to the walls of the blood vessel as a result of a wound or surgical procedure. It can also be caused by diseases of the blood vessel wall, whether through infection or malignancy. Diseases such as hemophilia, when the coagulation time of blood is delayed, can also cause hemorrhage.

Hemorrhages could be from different sources, which must be identified by the nurse for immediate intervention. When the arterial blood vessel is involved, the blood is bright red and escapes from the wound with pressure from a part closest to the heart.

Venous bleeding is characterized by dark red blood that flows steadily from the wound without pressure and far away from the heart. Capillary bleeding occurs in superficial layers of the skin, such as a scratch, and blood oozes from the wound, which is neither bright nor dark red.

The time for hemorrhage is also an important factor because bleeding might occur immediately after a vessel is damaged or days after damage (most likely due to an infection after a surgical procedure).

CNAs are expected to assess:

The skin: Loss of blood affects the skin, as it becomes pale, cold, and moist to the touch. Body temperature is also likely to decrease with bleeding.

The pulse: The pulse is rapid and weak. Depending on how severe the bleeding is, there is usually lowered blood volume and pressure.

The patient's facial expressions: The patient might appear anxious or afraid. The CNA is expected to relieve their fears and provide all necessary support.

Thirst: Loss of fluid associated with bleeding can result in thirst, hence the need to administer intravenous fluids to prevent dehydration.

Bleeding effects on the brain: Symptoms such as blurred vision, mental confusion, and unconsciousness can be indicators of various conditions, including significant blood loss. These symptoms can also be caused by other factors such as neurological issues, dehydration, or other medical conditions.

The pulse rate: During blood loss, the pulse is usually rapid and weak, depending on the severity of the hemorrhage.

The respiration rate: The respiration rate can increase in response to significant blood loss as the body attempts to compensate for decreased oxygen carrying capacity. However, gasping is not a usual response specifically to arterial blood loss. Gasping can occur in various critical conditions, such as cardiac arrest or severe respiratory distress.

Nursing interventions for general hemorrhage

- To arrest bleeding, apply pressure with the tips of the finger.
- Provide the patient with adequate rest.
- Reassure the patient.

- Raise the lower end of the bed to help blood flow by gravity to the brain if necessary. This may prevent unconsciousness.
- Assist the patient to breathe comfortably by removing tight clothing.
- Administer pain relief medications and intravenous fluids as prescribed.
- External wounds should be dressed and covered.
- Apply digital pressure at the site of bleeding in case it is an arterial blood vessel.
- For certain hemorrhages, such as epistaxis, hemoptysis, hematemesis, tooth socket bleeding, melena, and hematuria, intervention is made based on the specific conditions. However, the first point of action is always to investigate the cause of bleeding and arrest it as quickly as possible.

Burns

CNAs help manage patients with traumatic wounds such as burns. They must be familiar with the different procedures to suitably handle traumatic situations. This is because the management of traumatic wounds does not only involve medical attention but also a psychological examination of the casualty, with consideration for the relatives' response to the situation.

At all levels of care, CNAs begin with an assessment of the burn injury, which should be a repeated action to prevent complications. Patients are diagnosed afterward, and care is planned by the burn specialist and the nurse practitioner. Diagnoses often reported are related to inhalation, impaired respiratory function, altered vascular processes, skin damage, severe pain, mental dysfunctions, etc.

For example, if a man is brought into the emergency room of the hospital on a report of a fire accident, the nurse may assess and diagnose the patient to have a distorted breathing pattern due to the possible inflammation of the respiratory organs caused by inhalation. It might also be reported that the patient has severe abdominal and facial burns.

CNAs assist with oxygen administration as ordered by the physician and monitor breathing patterns regularly. It's also vital to suction patients, ensure that radiology tests are carried out, check respiratory rates and counts, assess sputum characteristics, etc.

The nurse administers analgesics and intravenous fluids and observes patient responses to the prescriptions. There is also a necessity to monitor heart rates and blood pressure and reassure clients as often as possible. To care for wounds after a surgical intervention such as skin grafting, CNAs assess the site for risk for infection, monitor fluid intake and output, check the wound drainage bag, and dress the wound as ordered.

There exists a possibility of impaired movement due to the splinting and immobilization requirements after the skin graft. CNAs help to elevate the upper and lower extremities and emphasize the importance of exercise and body movements. In cases where the burn occurred around the facial region, the client might be extremely depressed and traumatized. Even after wounds are cleaned to prevent infections, CNAs should also look out for the client's mental function, which could be impaired after a traumatic occurrence.

Patients with disabilities and skin damage after trauma are often referred for psychiatric consultations and rehabilitation to enable them to cope with the new condition. Relatives and caregivers must be educated by CNAs and assisted to understand experiences, reactions, and methods of coping with the situation.

Chapter 5: Specialized Care

One of the primary jobs of a CNA is to provide care for specialized patients and patients. This type of care may require an extra level of skill, dedication, and patience. These types of patients have needs that are different from other regular patients, and this puts them at risk of complications if they are not properly cared for.

These patients may have physical, psychological, mental, and emotional problems. It is the job of a CNA to be able to recognize and identify these types of patients and be knowledgeable about their conditions and how to care for them.

Physical Problems

Patients with physical problems may have impairments and disabilities of the eyes, ears, legs, and even internal organs. This can cause patients to be bedridden and in pain. It may also cause them to depend on CNAs and family members to bathe, go to the toilet, and eat.

Therefore, a CNA should know how to attend to patients with different physical problems and impairments. Some common physical problems will be discussed below, along with the management approach for each of these conditions.

Common Physical Impairments and Related Care

Sensory Impairment

The five senses of sight (eyes), hearing (ears), touch (hands), smell (nose), and taste (taste buds) help people understand and interact with the world. Sensory impairment occurs when an individual loses one or more of their senses or is overwhelmed by too much or too little sensory input. When a patient experiences sensory impairment, their ability to function safely is affected.

CNAs recognize patients' sensory problems and use strategies and resources to help improve their safety, function, quality of life, and overall well-being.

In an intact nervous system, sensory information from the environment is first received by sensory receptors, then transmitted to the brain, which processes the information and triggers a response in the body. When neurons send these messages to the body, they are called action potentials.

A sensory receptor perceives a stimulus and changes the sensation into an electrical signal that is sent to the brain for processing. The brain then sends a response signal to the appropriate part of the body. For example, if a pain receptor senses that a hand touches a hot tray, the pain signal is sent to the brain, where it can be interpreted. The brain then sends a signal to the hand, which prompts it to quickly pull back from the hot tray.

Sensory impairments can be any form of difficulty with one of the five senses. Loss of one of the senses, such as visual perception, can alter the way humans interact with the environment. For instance, when a person gradually loses their visual field, their ability to rely on other senses for information is likely to be increased.

Safety is always a top priority for patients with sensory impairment. Sometimes they need special devices to augment their impaired sense. For example, a patient who has impaired hearing may need a hearing aid.

Visual Impairment: Visual impairment is common in the elderly for various reasons. Older patients may have presbyopia, cataracts, and glaucoma. Other visual problems are astigmatism and macular degeneration.

In some individuals, cataracts, which are a discolored layer of the eye's lens, may develop. A person's eye may be visually impaired by a cloudiness of the pupil.

Hearing Impairment: A third of people over the age of 70 have hearing loss. Hearing is dependent on several things that turn sound waves in the air into electrical impulses. Hearing loss, also known as presbycusis, develops gradually in most people as they get older. It can become difficult to hear high-pitched sounds, which may include aspects of normal conversation, especially in the presence of loud background noise.

Hearing aids are often used to improve hearing in these types of patients. Although the cost of hearing aids can vary, it is important for patients and caregivers to take care of them and keep them in a safe place to prevent loss or damage. If a CNA is not sure how to put a hearing aid in a patient's ear, they should ask the nurse for help. A hearing aid can fit right in the ear or over the top.

Tinnitus is a medical term used to describe ringing in the ears. Certain medications like high doses of aspirin, antibiotics and certain diuretics can have ototoxic effects, which can potentially cause hearing loss or tinnitus.

Impairment in Feeling: Peripheral neuropathy is a disease that can make the nerves lose their ability to pick up sensations in parts of the body, especially the limbs. This loss of sensation may be due to touch, pressure, or vibration. It can pose a big risk to movement and coordination in the person. Peripheral neuropathy can be caused by a variety of factors, including diabetes mellitus, certain medications, traumatic injuries, infections, and nutritional deficiencies.

Speech Impairment

Aphasia is the most common type of speech impairment. It can be caused by a stroke or by injuries to certain areas of the brain. The injuries can make it difficult to form words and understand conversations. The terms 'expressive' and 'receptive' describe types of aphasia. Expressive aphasia involves difficulty in producing language, while receptive aphasia involves difficulty in understanding language. This means that patients may have difficulty speaking (expressive) and understanding (receptive).

Aphasia can lead to a lot of frustration. We've all tried to remember a word when it just doesn't come to mind. Imagine what it would be like to have to struggle every time you tried to talk to someone. Just as hearing loss can lead to isolation, patients with aphasia may become withdrawn, avoid social situations, or become angry and even violent if they aren't treated appropriately.

When a CNA works with patients with a speech disorder, one of the first interventions is to give them more time to formulate words or process what was said to them. Feeling rushed can worsen aphasia, so it's important to give patients plenty of opportunity to process and react. Writing conversations down on a board can also be beneficial, based on the person's cognitive abilities.

A speech-language pathologist evaluates patients with aphasia and develops a communication plan, which may include tools like a communication book with pictures or phrases to aid in communication, which are tailored to the patient's specific needs and abilities.

Changes in Mobility

A change in movement or mobility may be a short-term, long-term, or more permanent issue. When this occurs, it creates a complex healthcare issue that necessitates the involvement of multiple healthcare professionals. In reality, some degree of inactivity is common in most conditions, including strokes, leg fractures, multiple sclerosis, traumas, and obesity.

The capacity of a patient to alter and regulate their body posture is referred to as mobility. Physical mobility necessitates adequate muscular strength and energy, as well as appropriate skeletal stability, joint function, and neural synchronization. Functional mobility involves the capacity of the patient to navigate their environment, such as walk, stand from a chair, stand from a seated position, sit from a standing position, and maneuver.

Obesity has been linked to various health issues. Obesity can cause decreased mobility and increased risk of conditions like arthritis and cardiovascular disease. This can lead to impairments in physical activities of daily living, such as someone's ability to walk short distances, ascend stairs, and engage in activities such as showering. Age is the leading risk factor for impaired mobility, which leads to increased risk of disease and death in this population. Improved mobility also improves patients' quality of life and reduces caregiver and healthcare costs.

Paralysis is a loss of muscle function in a part of your body. It can be caused by damage to the nerves that control the muscles or to the spinal cord itself. It can affect any part of your body at any time in your life.

The signs and symptoms of paralysis are self-evident. When a person experiences paralysis, they will experience a loss of function in one or more areas of their body. In some cases, the onset of paralysis may be preceded by a sensation of tingling or numbness. Paralysis may be localized to one area of the face and body, or it may be generalized to every part of the body.

Changes in Elimination

The body removes waste products via the urinary tract and the gastrointestinal tract. Nurses and CNAs treat patients with common elimination challenges, including UTIs, uterine retention, constipation, diarrhea, and bowel incontinence.

The Urinary System

The urinary system is made up of the kidneys, ureters, bladder, and urethra. The kidneys filter blood to produce urine, which passes through the ureters to the bladder, where it is stored until it is excreted through the urethra. Its function is to remove waste from the body and control blood volume, blood pressure, electrolyte and metabolite levels, and blood pH. The kidneys filter blood through the nephrons. They also remove waste through urine. Urine leaves the kidneys through the ureters and enters the bladder, where it is stored until it is excreted (voided).

Some common conditions associated with elimination in the urinary system include:

- **Polyuria**: Polyuria is an excessive amount of urine output—over 2.5 L per 24 hours. Nocturia refers specifically to excessive urination at night, and it is distinct from polyuria, which is excessive urine output over 24 hours. Patients with nocturia may not necessarily experience polyuria, and vice versa. Common causes of polyuria include excessive fluid consumption, diuretic medication use, kidney disease, psychogenic polydipsia, diabetes mellitus, and diabetes insipidus. Anemia is not usually a cause of polyuria.
- **Oliguria**: This is defined as less than 400 ml of urine output over 24 hours. It is a condition in which urinary output is below the normal range. The most common underlying causes for oliguria are inadequate renal blood circulation, renal impairment, inadequate fluid intake, and dehydration.
- Other urinary elimination pathologies include hematuria, dysuria, urinary incontinence, and pyuria.

The Gastrointestinal System

The gastrointestinal system is made up of the mouth, the esophageal system, the stomach, the small intestine, the large intestine, and the anus. Food and liquid that has been digested passes through the digestive tract through peristalsis, which is the contraction and relaxation of muscles that creates wave-like bowel movements. The stomach breaks down food and liquid into digestive enzymes and empties into the small intestine. The small intestine muscles then mix the food and enzymes with bile from the pancreas and liver and push the mix forward for digestion.

Since healthy bowel and urination patterns differ from patient to patient, the treatment may be different for each patient group. Nurses must help patients with healthy elimination patterns and ensure they have regular soft bowel movements and adequate urination, as well as identify abnormal patterns (flatulence, constipation, diastasis, diarrhea, incontinence, fecal impaction, hemorrhoids).

Some of the pathologies in the gastrointestinal tract include:

- **Black stools:** Black stools are a common side effect of iron supplements or Pepto-Bismol, which contains bismuth.

- **Hematochezia**: This is also known as rectal bleeding. It is a type of bleeding that occurs in the lower gastrointestinal tract and is characterized by bright red blood in the stools. Rectal bleeding can vary in severity, ranging from minor bloodstains on toilet paper, which may be caused by conditions like hemorrhoids, to more extensive bleeding that could indicate a more serious condition and may require emergency care. However, not all minor bloodstains are due to hemorrhoids, and other causes should also be considered.

- **Tarry stools**: Melena is a type of stool that is characterized by a dark, sticky, and tar-like texture. This color is because the blood is from the upper gastrointestinal tract.

- **Constipation** is a reduction in passing feces or a reduction in bowel movement.

- **Diarrhea**: Diarrhea is characterized by three or more watery, loose stools within a 24-hour period.

- **Fecal impaction**: Fecal impaction refers to the accumulation of hardened feces in the rectum or lower part of the large intestine. It can cause difficulty in passing stools and may require medical intervention. It can be caused by certain medications, as well as secondary to obstructive conditions such as constipation.

Changes in Nutritional Needs

The nutritional needs of a patient may change as the patient ages and has problems with the gastrointestinal tract. In hospitals and other long-term care settings, the dietician evaluates patients regularly to determine their nutritional and fluid requirements. However, in group homes, assisted living, and home health settings, CNAs are often responsible for meal preparation. Knowledge of basic nutritional concepts will help them address a patient's nutritional needs.

Macronutrients: Macronutrients are a major component of a person's diet, providing energy and essential nutrients. These macronutrients are composed of carbohydrates, proteins, and fats. Insufficient amounts of the right nutrients in the diet can lead to health issues.

Excessive intake of macronutrients without adequate physical activity can result in cardiovascular disease, diabetes, kidney problems, and other chronic conditions. Conversely, inadequate macronutrient intake can lead to nutrient deficiencies and malnutrition.

The normal fluid needs of an average adult range from about 2 to 3 liters per day, depending on factors such as age, sex, weight, and the level of physical activity. A reduction in the output or input could cause dehydration. Some symptoms of dehydration include a dry mouth, sunken eyeballs, loss of skin turgor, and reduced urine output.

There are a variety of assistive devices available that facilitate the process of feeding patients. Some include built-up handles, weighted silverware, swivel spoons, covered cups, and plate guards.

Respiratory Problems

If you try to hold your breath for too long, your body's nervous system will kick in and start breathing again. That's because the cells need to make sure they use oxygen properly and do not release too much carbon dioxide.

Carbon dioxide buildup triggers the need to breathe, but the primary function of breathing is to obtain oxygen, which is critical for cellular function. Both the need to expel carbon dioxide and the need for oxygen are important factors driving respiration. The main parts of the lungs provide oxygen to the body's cells, get rid of the carbon dioxide that's left behind, and keep the pH balanced.

As the body gets older, the strength in the chest muscles weakens, and the small airways in the lungs, called the bronchioles, lose their flexibility and can break down. Age-related changes reduce an older adult's ability to breathe oxygen, which can lead to fatigue and difficulty in completing everyday tasks.

Some common respiratory problems include:

- **Asthma**: This is an inflammation and narrowing of the airways that is caused by various triggers, such as allergens and irritants. Asthma is not classified as a chronic obstructive pulmonary disease (COPD), but rather as a separate chronic inflammatory disease of the airways. The symptoms include coughing, wheezing, chest pain, breathing difficulties, and shortness of breath. It is the responsibility of the CNA to try to keep the patient at ease during an asthma attack and immediately report any breathing issues.

- **Bronchitis**: This is an inflammation of the bronchioles and may be acute or chronic. The symptoms may include a productive cough with mucus, fatigue, and chest discomfort. CNAs must position the patient appropriately to breathe well and encourage fluids to thin the mucus.

- **Chronic obstructive pulmonary disease**: These are lung diseases characterized by chronic airflow obstruction, which are mainly caused by smoking and other environmental factors. COPD includes chronic bronchitis and emphysema. The clinical features may include labored breathing, shortness of breath, and cyanosis. CNAs can encourage patients to quit smoking and encourage weight loss.

- **Lung cancer**: This is a malignant proliferation of cells in the lungs. The symptoms may include a chronic cough that is productive of blood, chest pain, and shortness of breath. CNAs can position the patient to breathe well, counsel smoking cessation, and advise lifestyle modification.

Part of the responsibility of a CNA is to care for patients on oxygen. This may involve restricting smoking in the room where oxygen is being used. Also, the patient should be positioned appropriately and assisted to use the oxygen device as needed. CNAs may also educate patients on how to use devices like oxygen concentrators.

Changes in Skin Integrity

The skin is made up of three different layers: the epidermis, dermis, and hypodermis. The skin is made up of oils, fats, blood vessels, the hair, and the hair shaft. The skin is not only important for thermoregulation but also helps in the exchange of body fluids.

However, as people age, the components of the skin change. For example, older patients have a reduced amount of fat in the skin, so they may have problems controlling their body temperature.

Also, some patients have reduced oils and sweat production, so it is important for them to have less frequent baths. They may have partial body baths instead of full-body baths.

CNAs should observe a client's feet and report any concerns and nail care for diabetic patients can be safely performed by trained CNAs. Diabetic patients have a heightened risk of foot problems, so careful monitoring and appropriate care are essential.

Pain Management

Pain is a physiological response that motivates the body to avoid potentially hazardous situations, such as a hot pan. It also serves to remind the body to safeguard an injured area as it heals. For example, pain might prevent a patient from walking on an injured ankle.

Generally, pain is resolved after the stimulus that caused the injury has been removed, and the patient's body has healed. Additionally, pain can occur when there is no identifiable stimulus, harm, or illness.

There are two types of pain:

- Acute.
- Chronic.

Acute pain lasts for just a short time. As the body heals, the pain should subside.

Chronic pain, on the other hand, is a long-term condition that persists for more than six months. It can have a significant impact on an individual's psychological, social, and behavioral functions, as well as their daily activities. Common chronic medical conditions include osteoarthritis, spinal conditions, and fibromyalgia, as well as peripheral neuropathy.

The primary role of CNAs is to assess the level of pain in a patient, report the pain to the nurses, and provide other forms of comfort aside from analgesics.

Provide for the Safety, Care, and Comfort of Patients with Physical Impairments

CNAs also care for patients with physical disabilities. It is important to not only care for these individuals but make them comfortable. Personal caregiving involves assistance with tasks that a patient is unable to do on their own.

Don't assume a patient needs help. Instead, offer help and wait for them to say yes. If they say yes, wait for them to give you instructions. You may also ask them what you can do for them. Make sure you respect their response.

Impact of Impairments on Patient Safety, Care, and Comfort

Patient comfort isn't just about pain and symptom management. Patients should be comfortable in their environment, spiritually connected, surrounded by family, receive timely support, participate in the treatment plan, and engage with dedicated staff. Research shows that patient comfort directly impacts the overall patient experience.

Some common causes of impairment to a patient's safety and comfort include:

- Pain.
- Stress.
- Physical disability.
- Chronic disease.

Patients may verbalize the pain, feel worried, or be in distress. They may be irritable and may have rapid breathing. All of this may affect the prognosis of the treatment and the psychology of the patient. These impairments may cause mental and behavioral disorders and even learning challenges for some patients.

Psychological Problems

The definition of health, per the World Health Organization, includes the psychology of the patient. Poor psychological and mental health can lead to impairments. CNAs need to understand how to manage these impairments within their scope of responsibilities.

Common Psychological Impairments and Related Care

A person with a psychological disorder has an illness that affects the person's thinking, emotions, or behavior and increases their chances of disability, pain, death, or loss of independence.

Some common psychological impairments include:

- **Bipolar disorder**: Bipolar disorder isn't just about mood swings. It's also about changes in activity and energy levels. People with bipolar disorder often experience periods of high and low moods.

  Mania is a time of elevated emotions, with lots of activity and energy. During this period, patients feel the need to engage in a lot of activities, and they usually have a lot of energy.

  The episodes are characterized by a clinically significant decline in mood and functioning, which goes beyond typical sadness or a lack of enthusiasm. Depressive episodes in bipolar disorder can include a range of symptoms such as pervasive low mood, a significant loss of interest or pleasure in almost all activities, significant weight loss or gain, insomnia or hypersomnia, fatigue or loss of energy, feelings of worthlessness or excessive or inappropriate guilt, diminished ability to think or concentrate, and recurrent thoughts of death or suicide. These episodes are more severe and enduring than ordinary fluctuations in mood and can significantly impair a person's daily life.

- **Neurodevelopmental disorders:** Neurodevelopmental diseases are those that are diagnosed in infancy, childhood, or later in life. Autism and attention deficit hyperactivity disorder (ADHD) are examples.

  Patients with ADHD have clinical features like hyperactivity and impulsiveness. They find it difficult to pay attention for a long time, and this affects their work and daily life.

  Autistic patients have impaired forms of communication and social interactions. They may have behavioral changes that make it difficult for them to cope with others.

- **Anxiety**: Patients may have prolonged feelings of fear and could suffer behavioral changes. They may also have impaired social interactions with their friends and peers. Some patients have specific fears or phobias for conditions like heights and animals like snakes or spiders. Others may have a persistent form of anxiety toward everyday life and activities.

- **Trauma**: Trauma can lead to anxiety and psychological disorders. A form of this is called post-traumatic stress disorder (PTSD). In this condition, patients have anxiety after a traumatic situation, such as the death of a loved one or a car accident. Symptoms of PTSD may include episodes of recollection or re-enactment of the event.

- Other common psychological problems include narcolepsy, insomnia, anorexia nervosa, and panic disorders.

Special Considerations for the Safety, Care, and Comfort of Patients with Psychological Impairments

Patients with psychological problems need special consideration and care. Some of the approaches may include reorientation of the patient as often as necessary to person, location, and time.

A patient's inability to retain reality orientation can lead to distress or exacerbation of confusion. Repeated reorientation enables the patient to gain a sense of autonomy and establishes a relationship of trust with the healthcare provider.

It is essential to take the patient's safety into account at all times, as mental health issues can influence response to external stimuli.

Appropriate safety precautions may include the implementation of side rails, close monitoring, or seizure precautions, as indicated.

Patients with mental health issues may act out impulsively if they're overstimulated, so a quiet environment must be maintained.

Care for Dying Patients and Postmortem Care

CNAs also have to care for patients who are dying and provide postmortem care. The care of a dying patient may also be called end-of-life care. In this type of care, the patient and family members both need to be attended to.

Grief Process

Grief helps in the resolution of the emotional distress caused by the loss of a loved one. It is also important in the healing process of individuals.

Elisabeth Kübler-Ross originally described these stages (denial, anger, bargaining, depression, and acceptance) in her book "On Death and Dying" as part of the dying process. Grief is a highly individual process and can vary widely in its expression and progression. People may not experience all these stages or may go through them in a different order. The stages of grief have evolved in understanding and are now more commonly viewed as overlapping and cyclical, rather than a linear progression.

- **Shock:** This is a state of numb disbelief in response to the news of the death of a loved one.
- **Denial**: Denial involves not accepting the loss of a loved one or the feelings associated with it.
- **Anger**: During this phase, a person may vent their grievances against the deceased person, medical professionals, or relatives.

- **Bargaining**: Bargaining can occur at any point in the grieving process. The grieving person feels guilt in this stage.

- **Depression**: There is a feeling of emptiness and profound sorrow. It may also involve a withdrawal from everyday activities and previously enjoyed activities.

- **Acceptance**: Acceptance is about acknowledging and accepting the reality of the loss. It means understanding that the loss is permanent and coming to terms with it.

Respond to the Emotional Needs of the Patient, other Patients, Family, and Caregivers in the Grief Process

The loss of a loved one, whether it be a spouse, sibling, or friend, can be a difficult and overwhelming experience for any patient. Caregivers and CNAs must be available to provide support and guidance throughout the grieving process, which can manifest in a variety of ways, such as emotional breakdowns, anger, or feelings of isolation.

Some people don't go through all the stages of grief. It is important to note these types of people and help them. Here are some of the ways CNAs can help:

- Listen.

- Don't force patients to share their feelings. Some of them may not want to talk about their loss.

- Give patients a safe space to share their feelings and grief.

- Offer support and volunteer to help in any way.

Factors that Influence Responses to Grief

People grieve differently. Some of the factors that may determine how people grieve include culture, past experience, and religion.

People who are close to each other often find it difficult to accept the death of the other person. But if the death of the deceased has been anticipated, perhaps due to a chronic illness, the death may be more bearable.

Physical Changes and Needs as Death Approaches

As the end of life approaches, people may become less interested in the outside world and day-to-day activities. This may lead to a decrease in social activities, as well as a desire to maintain only a small group of friends.

As the person nears the end of life, they may say they see or hear others who have gone before them, and caregivers may hear them talking with a deceased friend or relative. This particular communication can be worrisome for those who care for the person. Denying the experience can be a difficult and frustrating experience for the person.

Patients may also experience delirium, a condition in which a person is not aware of their surroundings. It may be caused by a single factor or by a combination of factors, such as medication or changes in metabolism. Symptoms may include agitation, hallucination, and a fluctuation in levels of consciousness. Generally, these symptoms can be managed with medication. Patients may also experience appetite changes, breathing changes, and changes in body temperature.

Postmortem Care Procedures

The nurse will assess the time of a patient's death and adhere to agency regulations. If family members are present, they should be allowed to remain with the body for as long as is necessary for them to say their goodbyes. If they have any religious or cultural customs, they should be allowed to express them. For instance, people from certain cultures may prefer to wash their loved one's body after death. The CNA will then prepare the body for transportation.

It is important to respect the wishes and customs of the family regarding their presence during postmortem care. Families may have cultural, religious, or personal preferences about being with their loved one during this time. The patient should be given a bed bath and then positioned properly. After the bath, a fresh gown should be provided. The patient's eyelids should be gently closed, and a rolled towel should be placed under the chin to stabilize the jaw. Clean linens should be used to cover the face and head of the patient. It is important to check facility policy for the application of an identification bracelet.

The exam will test you to ensure you know each of the following steps for standard nursing procedures.

Chapter 6: Skill Tests

Skill 1

Handwashing

1. Appropriately introduce yourself and address the client by name.
2. Turn on the faucet.
3. Wet your hands and wrists meticulously.
4. Apply soap to your hands.
5. Lather your wrists, hands, and fingers.
6. Keep your hands higher than your elbows during the washing process. This position ensures that water flows from the cleanest area (your hands) to the less clean area (your elbows) and prevents contaminated water from moving back towards your hands.
7. To clean all fingernails, press your fingertips against the palm of the opposite hand.
8. Correctly use clean, dry towels to remove moisture from your hands. This process should start from the fingertips.
9. Appropriately dispose of towels in the waste bin.
10. Turn off the faucet with dry, clean paper towels, which you then dispose of.
11. Do not make any form of contact with the inside of the sink the entire time.

Skill 2

Apply Knee-high Elastic Stockings

1. Provide a clear and simple explanation of the procedure to the client.
2. Maintain eye contact with appropriate verbal and nonverbal cues.
3. Use a door, curtain, or privacy screen, as appropriate.
4. Make sure a signaling device is close at hand.
5. Place the patient in a supine position during the application of the stocking.
6. Place the foot of the stocking over the client's toes, foot, and heel.
7. Pull the top of the stocking over the foot, heel, and toes.
8. Move the patient's foot and leg naturally and ensure the limbs and joints are not overextended.
9. The procedure must be completed without creases in the stocking, and the heel and toe of the stocking should be appropriately placed.
10. If the procedure is carried out on a mannequin, the stocking should be crease-free.
11. Wash your hands after the procedure.

Skill 3

Assist with Ambulation and use a Transfer Belt

1. Provide a simple, clear explanation of the procedure and maintain eye contact.
2. Use a door, curtain, or privacy screen, as appropriate.
3. Place a signaling device within reach.
4. Ensure that the client is in nonskid shoes or footwear before you help them to stand.
5. Ensure that the bed is at an appropriate, safe level for the patient.
6. Ensure that the client is seated in the right position with their feet placed flat on the floor.
7. Apply the transfer belt securely at the waist right above the client's clothing.
8. Tell the patient what to do before you help the patient stand. Part of the information conveyed must include a prearranged signal to let the patient know when it is time to stand.
9. When assisting with ambulation using a transfer belt, the caregiver should stand slightly to the side and slightly behind the client, not directly in front. This position provides better support and stability for the client during standing and walking, and allows the caregiver to guide and control movement more effectively.
10. Stand knee-to-knee or toe-to-toe with the client to help maintain stability.
11. To assist the client to stand, hold the transfer belt on the two sides with an upward-facing grasp.
12. Walk just behind the client on either the left or right side while you grasp the belt.
13. Help the client get to the bed and remove the transfer belt.
14. Wash your hands after the procedure.

Skill 4

Assist with a Bedpan

The proper procedure to assist a patient to use a bedpan is:

1. Describe the procedure to the client with constant face-to-face interaction and speak in a slow, clear, and direct manner.
2. Use a door, curtain, or privacy screen, as appropriate.
3. Place a signaling device within reach.
4. The head of the bed should be properly lowered before the bedpan is placed.
5. Before the bedpan is placed, put on clean gloves.
6. The client's buttocks must sit well on the bedpan.
7. Dispose of your gloves in a waste bin and make sure not to contaminate yourself.
8. The head of the bed should be raised after the gloves have been disposed of. Ensure the client is positioned well.
9. Toilet paper should always be within arm's reach.
10. Handwipes should also be close by, where they can be used by clients when a session is over.
11. Put on clean gloves and lower the head of the bed before you remove the bedpan.
12. Properly cover the client.
13. Completely empty the bedpan into a toilet and rinse it.
14. Place the empty bedpan in its designated spot in the room.
15. Dispose of your gloves carefully.
16. Wash your hands.

Skill 5

Clean a Client's Dentures

1. Put your gloves on.
2. Partially fill the sink with water.
3. Line the sink with a liner.
4. Thoroughly rinse the dentures in moderate-temperature running water.
5. Apply toothpaste to the toothbrush.
6. Properly brush all surfaces of the dentures.
7. Use warm running water to rinse the dentures after you wash them. Rinse the toothbrush too.
8. Wash the dentures' lid and cup.
9. It is recommended to put the cleaned dentures in a denture cup filled with cool or room-temperature water or a denture-soaking solution. Using hot or warm water can potentially warp the dentures, especially if they are made of certain types of materials.
10. Cover the cup with the dentures' lid.
11. Place the rinsed toothbrush in its designated spot.
12. Throw the sink liner away and drain the sink.
13. Remove and throw away the gloves. Be careful not to contaminate yourself.

Skill 6

Record a Client's Radial Pulse

1. Describe the steps in the procedure to the client with a constant face-to-face interaction. Make sure your words are spoken in a slow, clear, and direct manner.
2. Wash your hands.
3. Locate the radial pulse with your fingers on the wrist of the client.
4. Beats should be counted over the span of a minute.
5. Make sure a signaling device is within reach of the patient.
6. You should record the pulse rate within plus or minus four beats of the evaluator's reading.

Skill 7

Count and Record a Client's Respiration Cycles

1. Describe the steps in the procedure to the client with a constant face-to-face interaction. Make sure your words are spoken in a slow, clear, and direct manner.
2. Respiration counts should be done within the time span of a minute.
3. Make sure a signaling device is always close to the patient.
4. Ensure your hands are thoroughly washed before the procedure.
5. Your reading should be within plus or minus two breaths of what the evaluator records.

Skill 8

Put on and Remove PPE

1. Select a gown and then unfold it.
2. Position the back of the gown toward you, then place your arms through the sleeves.
3. Secure the opening at the neck of the gown.
4. Fasten the waist of the gown and make sure that the back of the gown is properly covered.
5. Put on clean gloves.
6. The cuffs of the gloves should extend over the cuffs of the gown.
7. Gloves should be removed with the opposite gloved hand before the gown is removed. To remove the other gloved hand, slip your fingers (from the ungloved hands) into the cuff of the glove and evert it.
8. The gloves should be disposed of in a trash container. Make sure you avoid contamination during this process.
9. Untie the gown at the neck and waist area.
10. Turn the gown wrong-side-out as you remove it.
11. The gown should be disposed of in a trash container. Make sure you avoid contamination during this process.
12. After the procedure, wash your hands thoroughly.

Skill 9

Clothe Clients with an Affected Right Arm

1. Describe the steps in the procedure to the client with a constant face-to-face interaction. Speak in a slow, clear, and direct manner.
2. Use a door, curtain, or privacy screen, as appropriate.
3. Place a signaling device within reach.
4. Angle the bed in a low position.
5. Ask the client about the choice of shirt they would like to wear.
6. The client's body should not be overexposed.
7. When dressing a client with an affected right arm, you should start by placing the affected arm (right arm) into the sleeve first, followed by the unaffected arm (left arm). This approach minimizes movement and discomfort for the client.
8. Be cautious as you place the right (affected) arm into the right sleeve of the shirt and then the left.
9. The limbs and joints of the client should be carefully handled. The client's body must be manipulated gently and should not be over-stretched.
10. The clothing must be in place and correctly positioned.
11. After the procedure, wash your hands thoroughly.

Skill 10

Assist Clients who Cannot Feed Themselves

1. Describe the steps in the procedure to the client with a constant face-to-face interaction. Make sure your words are spoken in a slow, clear, and direct manner.
2. Before you feed a client, ask for their name and then compare it with the name card on the food tray.
3. The client must be seated in an upright position, which is usually 75 to 90 degrees.
4. Place a signaling device within reach.
5. The tray should be placed in such a way that the client can easily see it.
6. The client's hands should be properly washed before the meal.
7. Sit directly in front of the client.
8. Inform the client about the food or beverage available on the tray.
9. Ask the client for their first choice of meal.
10. Feed the client with a spoon. Offer a variety of food items from the tray, while respecting the client's preferences and dietary restrictions. Inform the client about the contents of each spoonful before feeding.
11. Beverages should be offered to the client at least once during meals.
12. Ask for the client's consent before feeding the next round of the meal.
13. The client's mouth and hands should be cleaned after the meal.
14. Remove the food tray.
15. The client should still be seated in an upright position of 75 to 90 degrees after the meal.
16. After the procedure, wash your hands thoroughly.

Skill 11

Provide a Professional Bed Bath

1. Describe the steps in the procedure to the client with a constant face-to-face interaction. Make sure your words are spoken in a slow, clear, and direct manner.
2. Use a door, curtain, or privacy screen, as appropriate.
3. Take off the gown worn by the client and place it in the designated container. Make sure that the client's lower body and chest area are covered.
4. Place a signaling device within reach.
5. Angle the bed in a low position.
6. Confirm that the bath water's temperature is safe and comfortable for the client.
7. Put on clean gloves.
8. Start with the client's eyes. Wash them gently with a wet washcloth that contains no soap. After you wash all sections of the eyes, you can proceed to the face.
9. The face should be dried with a dry towel.
10. Gently lift the client's arm and wash it with a soapy washcloth. Be cautious to support the arm and avoid overextending the joints. After washing, place a towel underneath the arm to catch any drips.
11. Soap can now be applied to the washcloth.
12. Cover the rest of the client's body while you wash the fingers, fingernails, hands, armpits, and arms.
13. Wipe and dry the fingers and the other body parts that have been washed.
14. The limbs and joints of the client should be handled carefully. The body of the client must be manipulated gently and should not be over-stretched.
15. Provide a clean gown for the client.
16. Wash and dry the basin used.
17. The clean basin should be placed in its designated spot.
18. Dispose of the washcloth as appropriate.
19. The gloves used should be disposed of in a trash container. Make sure you avoid contamination during this process, and then wash your hands thoroughly.

Skill 12

Measure Urinary Output

1. Put on clean gloves before you pick up the bedpan.
2. Carefully pour the contents of the bedpan into the container. Make sure not to splash.
3. The container must be placed at eye level to measure the urine amount, which should be estimated to the nearest 25 ml/cc.
4. After the measurement process is over, dispose of the bedpan contents into a toilet and rinse the bedpan.
5. Wash the measurement container and pour the contents into a toilet.
6. The gloves used should be disposed of in a trash container. Make sure you avoid contamination during this process, and then wash your hands thoroughly. All this should be done before you record the output.
7. You should record the contents within plus or minus 25 ml/cc of what the evaluator recorded.

Skill 13

Record an Ambulatory Client's Weight

1. Describe the steps in the procedure to the client with a constant face-to-face interaction. Make sure your words are spoken in a slow, clear, and direct manner.
2. Clients should put on nonslip shoes before they step on the scale.
3. The scale should be set to zero before the client steps on it.
4. To obtain the client's weight, they must stand at the exact center of the scale.
5. Wash your hands before you record the client's weight.
6. After the process is over, ask the client to step off the scale.
7. The indicator on the scale determines the weight of the client. Your reading should be within plus or minus 0.9 kg of what the evaluator records.

Skill 14

Perform Passive Range of Motion (PROM) for One Knee and Ankle

1. Describe the steps in the procedure to the client with a constant face-to-face interaction. Make sure your words are spoken in a slow, clear, and direct manner.
2. Use a door, curtain, or privacy screen, as appropriate.
3. Place a signaling device within reach.
4. Angle the bed in a low position.
5. Ensure the client lies supine on the bed and ask them to give a sign if they feel pain or discomfort.
6. During the exercise, ensure you support the leg before you extend the knee and return it to the client's original position (flexion). Do this at least three times or less if pain is verbalized. Move the joint naturally and smoothly. The body of the client must be manipulated gently and should not be over-stretched. End all movements if the client complains of pain.
7. During this exercise process, ensure you support the foot close to the bed and push or pull the foot toward the head of the client (dorsiflexion). Push/pull the foot in a way that the toes point down (plantar flexion). Do this at least three times or less if the client complains of pain. The body of the client must be manipulated gently and should not be over-stretched. End all movements if the client complains of pain.
8. After the procedure, wash your hands thoroughly.

Skill 15

Perform PROM for a Single Shoulder

1. Describe the steps in the procedure to the client with a constant face-to-face interaction. Make sure your words are spoken in a slow, clear, and direct manner.
2. Use a door, curtain, or privacy screen, as appropriate.
3. Place a signaling device within reach.
4. Angle the bed in a low position.
5. The client must be asked to verbalize pain if it is felt at any point during the exercise.
6. During this exercise process, ensure you support the arm at the elbow and wrist. Raise the arm and stretch it towards the head or ear level, and then return it to the original position (extension). Do this at least three times or less if pain is verbalized. The client's body must be manipulated gently and should not be over-stretched. End all movements if the client complains of pain.
7. During this exercise process, ensure you support the arm at the elbow and wrist. Raise the arm to the side at shoulder level and then return it to the side of the body (abduction). Do this at least three times or less if pain is verbalized. The client's body must be manipulated gently and should not be over-stretched. End all movements if the client complains of pain.
8. After the procedure, wash your hands thoroughly.

Skill 16

Place the Client on their Side

1. Describe the steps in the procedure to the client with a constant face-to-face interaction. Make sure your words are spoken in a slow, clear, and direct manner.
2. Use a door, curtain, or privacy screen, as appropriate.
3. Place a signaling device within reach.
4. Lower the head of the bed.
5. Raise the rail on the side of the bed that the patient will be turned toward.
6. Assist the client to turn on their side toward the side rail.
7. Support the head of the client with a pillow.
8. Ensure that the arms and shoulders of the client are arranged so that the client is not lying on their arm.
9. The top arm should be assisted with a supportive device.
10. Place an assistive device at the back of the client.
11. Place an assistive device between the legs in such a way that the knees are flexed.
12. After the procedure, wash your hands thoroughly.

Skill 17

Provide Catheter Care

1. Describe the steps in the procedure to the client with a constant face-to-face interaction. Make sure your words are spoken in a slow, clear, and direct manner.
2. Use a door, curtain, or privacy screen, as appropriate.
3. Place a signaling device within reach.
4. Angle the bed in a low position.
5. Confirm that the bath water temperature is safe and comfortable for the client.
6. Put on clean gloves.
7. Put linen protectors under the client's buttocks.
8. Areas to be exposed shouldn't go beyond the hips and knees.
9. Add soap to the towel or washcloth.
10. The catheter should be held at the meatus. Do *not* tug. The catheter should be cleaned starting at the meatus and after moving outward four inches. Move in the opposite direction and use a new surface of the washcloth for each stroke.
11. The catheter should be rinsed unidirectionally four inches away from the meatus with a new surface of the washcloth used for each stroke.
12. The catheter should be dried at least four inches away from the meatus in a unidirectional fashion and with a different surface of a dry cloth used for each stroke.
13. The contents of the basin should be disposed of. Then, the basin should be washed, dried, and placed in its designated section.
14. Dispose of the washcloth and the linen protector into the designated waste container.
15. Make sure your clothing doesn't make contact with the washcloth.
16. Dispose of your gloves in a trash container. Make sure you avoid contamination during this process, and then wash your hands thoroughly.

Skill 18

Provide Foot Care for a Single Foot

1. Describe the steps in the procedure to the client with a constant face-to-face interaction. Make sure your words are spoken in a slow, clear, and direct manner.
2. Use a door, curtain, or privacy screen, as appropriate.
3. Place a signaling device within reach.
4. Confirm that the bath water temperature is safe and comfortable for the client.
5. The basin should be in a comfortable position for the client to use.
6. Put on clean gloves.
7. Place the client's bare foot into the water.
8. Add soap to the towel or washcloth.
9. Lift the client's foot from the water and wash it thoroughly, including between the toes.
10. The foot should be well rinsed, including the gaps between the toes.
11. Dry the foot with a towel, including in between the toes.
12. The top and bottom of the foot should be rubbed with lotion, excluding between the toes. Excess lotion should be wiped away with a dry towel.
13. Ensure the foot is supported during the process.
14. The contents of the basin should be disposed of. The basin should be washed and dried and placed in its designated spot.
15. Dispose of the washcloth as appropriate.
16. Dispose of your gloves in a trash container. Make sure you avoid contamination during this process, and then wash your hands thoroughly.

Skill 19

Provide Mouth Care

1. Describe the steps in the procedure to the client with a constant face-to-face interaction. Make sure your words are spoken in a slow, clear, and direct manner.
2. Use a door, curtain, or privacy screen, as appropriate.
3. Place a signaling device within reach.
4. Angle the bed in a low position.
5. The client should be properly seated (usually at 75 to 90 degrees) before any mouth care is provided.
6. Put on clean gloves.
7. A cloth towel should be placed across the client's chest before any mouth care is provided.
8. Have a readily available cup of water with a moistened toothbrush.
9. Apply toothpaste to the moistened toothbrush.
10. Every corner and surface of the mouth should be thoroughly brushed with gentle motions (this includes the tongue).
11. Place the basin close to the chin of the client. The client should then rinse their mouth.
12. Wipe the mouth of the client and remove the cloth used to cover their chest.
13. Dispose of the towel in a container.
14. The contents of the basin should be disposed of. The basin should be washed and dried. The brush should also be washed.
15. The gloves used should be disposed of in a trash container. Make sure you avoid contamination during this process, and then wash your hands thoroughly.

Skill 20

Provide Perineal Care

1. Describe the steps in the procedure to the client with a constant face-to-face interaction. Make sure your words are spoken in a slow, clear, and direct manner.
2. Use a door, curtain, or privacy screen, as appropriate.
3. Place a signaling device within reach.
4. Angle the bed in a low position.
5. Confirm that the bath water temperature is safe and comfortable for the client.
6. Put on clean gloves.
7. A cloth protector should be placed under the perineal area.
8. When you expose the perineal area, only expose the section between the hips and knees.
9. Add soap to the towel or washcloth.
10. For females, the genital area should be wiped from front to back. Use a new surface of the towel for each stroke. For males, clean the tip of the penis first, then the shaft, moving towards the scrotum, using a new surface of the towel for each stroke.
11. To rinse the soap in the genital area, a clean washcloth should be used. Wipe from front to back with a new surface of the towel used for each stroke.
12. Dry the genital area with a dry washcloth from front to back.
13. Turn the patient to the side.
14. Clean the rectal area after the genitals are washed. This area must be wiped from front to back with a new surface of the towel used for each stroke.
15. To rinse the soap in the rectal area, a clean washcloth should be used. Wipe from front to back with a new surface of the towel used for each stroke.
16. Dry the rectal area with a dry washcloth from front to back.
17. The client should be properly repositioned.
18. The contents of the basin should be disposed of. The basin should be washed and dried and placed in the designated section.
19. Dispose of the washcloth and the cloth protector into a container.
20. Make sure your clothing doesn’t make contact with the washcloth.
21. Dispose of your gloves in a trash container. Make sure you avoid contamination during this process, and then wash your hands thoroughly.

Skill 21

Use a Transfer Belt to Transfer a Client from a Bed to a Wheelchair

1. Describe the steps in the procedure to the client with a constant face-to-face interaction. Make sure your words are spoken in a slow, clear, and direct manner
2. Use a door, curtain, or privacy screen, as appropriate.
3. Place a signaling device within reach.
4. The wheelchair should be positioned close to the bed, with the head of the bed facing the foot or vice versa before you assist the client to stand.
5. Fold up or remove the footrest.
6. Lock the wheels of the wheelchair.
7. Lock the bed wheels.
8. The client should be seated with their feet flat on the ground and must wear shoes.
9. The transfer belt must be firmly applied at the waist over the client's clothing.
10. Provide instructions and prearranged signals to alert the client when it is time to stand.
11. Position yourself in front of the client. Say the signal—for instance, count to three to alert the client to stand.
12. On cue, assist the client. Hold the transfer belt on each side in an upward pull. To maintain the stance of the client's legs, stand either toe to toe or knee to knee with the client.
13. To assist the client to stand, place the back of their legs toward the wheelchair.
14. The client should be lowered toward the wheelchair.
15. The hips of the client should touch the back of the wheelchair while the transfer belt is removed.
16. Place the client's feet on the footrests.
17. After the procedure, wash your hands thoroughly.

Skill 22

Manually Measure a Client's Blood Pressure

1. Describe what you want to do with a constant face-to-face interaction. Make sure your words are spoken slowly, clearly, and directly.
2. Clean the diaphragm and earpiece of the stethoscope with alcohol.
3. The arm of the client should be positioned in such a way that the palm is up and the upper arm is exposed.
4. Search for the brachial artery in the inner part of the arm, close to the bend of the elbow.
5. The blood pressure cuff should be firmly placed over the client's upper arm, with the sensor placed over the brachial artery.
6. Put the earpiece of the stethoscope in your ears and the diaphragm on the area where the brachial artery pulsations can be picked out.
7. The cuff should be inflated to a level 20-30 mmHg above the level where the radial pulse disappears. If a beat is heard right after the cuff starts to deflate, deflate it completely, wait a few seconds, and then reinflate it to a slightly higher pressure.
8. The cuff should be deflated slowly. Take note of the first beat (systolic) and the last beat (diastolic). If estimation is needed, measurements are rounded up to the nearest 2 mmHg.
9. Remove the cuff.
10. Wash your hands thoroughly before recording.
11. You should record both systolic and diastolic pulse pressures within plus or minus 8 mmHg of what the examiner records.

Test 1: Questions

(1) Which of the following does a CNA not do?

(A) Assist patients with meals and toileting.

(B) Participate in patient-care discussions.

(C) Assist with patient transfer and repositioning.

(D) Delegate duties to other CNAs.

(2) A 45-year-old man is brought to the emergency department with sudden-onset difficulty with breathing. He is a known asthmatic patient who does not use his inhaler frequently. The healthcare setting where this patient is managed is a/an:

(A) Chronic care setting.

(B) Sub-acute setting.

(C) Acute care setting.

(D) General care setting.

(3) Which of the following acts would most likely violate a patient's right to confidentiality?

(A) A CNA reports a patient's vitals to the staff nurse.

(B) A CNA keeps the door open and discusses matters with a patient in a loud voice.

(C) A CNA walks by a room and does not greet a patient.

(D) A CNA forgets to escalate a patient's complaints to the staff nurse.

(4) CNA Tanya visits the room of a 55-year-old hearing-impaired patient. Which of the following is the correct communication approach?

(A) Sit directly in front of the patient to talk.

(B) Give the patient a note to read.

(C) Only speak with the patient's children.

(D) Speak through a megaphone.

(5) Which of the following diseases require airborne protective measures to prevent spread?

(A) Measles.

(B) Cholera.

(C) Typhoid.

(D) Malaria.

(6) A 55-year-old woman is brought to the emergency department with a cough, dyspnea, swollen legs, and distended neck veins. What is the most likely diagnosis?

(A) Myocardial infarction.

(B) Heart failure.

(C) Pneumothorax.

(D) Pneumonia.

(7) A 40-year-old victim of a car accident is brought to the emergency department in shock. Which vital signs are consistent with shock?

(A) Fast and thready pulse.

(B) Slow pulse.

(C) High blood pressure.

(D) Loud pulse.

(8) A 40-year-old man comes to the clinic for treatment of obesity. Which parameters are used to calculate BMI?

(A) Weight and mid-arm circumference.

(B) Weight and pulse rate.

(C) Weight and hip ratio.

(D) Weight and height.

(9) What is a possible complication of chronic constipation?

(A) Weight loss.

(B) Weight gain.

(C) Dehydration.

(D) Fecal impaction.

(10) Osteoporosis is a condition characterized by:

(A) Loss of bone tissue.

(B) Thickened bone.

(C) Broken bone.

(D) Bone shortening.

(11) An individual forgets or misplaces commonly used materials such as keys or eyeglasses. This is an example of memory loss found in:

(A) Dementia.

(B) Normal aging.

(C) Delirium.

(D) Challenging behavior.

(12) What is the primary purpose of using the Trendelenburg position for a patient?

(A) To reduce lower back pain.

(B) To facilitate breathing in patients with respiratory issues.

(C) To elevate the patient's feet higher than the head.

(D) To prepare the patient for abdominal surgery.

(13) A 70-year-old man develops an insidious onset of poor vision. The patient could see very well a decade ago, but now, objects appear blurry. Visual examination shows opacity of the lens. What is the diagnosis?

(A) Myopia.

(B) Hyperopia.

(C) Cataract.

(D) Astigmatism.

(14) Diarrhea refers to when a patient:

(A) Passes watery stool three or more times in a day.

(B) Passes watery stool three or more times a week.

(C) Passes watery stool once a year.

(D) Has an occasional episode of loose stool.

(15) A 66-year-old man with chronic obstructive pulmonary disease is managed at home. The patient's condition has worsened significantly in the last few years. The patient requires:

(A) Long-term oxygen therapy.

(B) Fluid therapy.

(C) Electrolyte therapy.

(D) Cough medications.

(16) Why would a CNA perform a random blood sugar test on a patient?
(A) To determine if the patient is hydrated.
(B) To check for the immediate blood sugar levels at any time.
(C) To check if lots of sugary foods have been eaten in the morning.
(D) To prepare for a surgical procedure.

(17) Which body parts should be protected during a bath to prevent irritation from shampoo?
(A) Nose.
(B) Ear.
(C) Eyes.
(D) Genitals.

(18) Mr. James, a 40-year-old man, is diagnosed with gastric cancer with gastric outlet obstruction. What is the most appropriate method to feed Mr. James?
(A) Oral.
(B) Nasogastric tube.
(C) Parenteral feeding.
(D) No feeding.

(19) Which class of food does glucose belong to?
(A) Carbohydrates.
(B) Proteins.
(C) Fats.
(D) Oils.

(20) All of the following are nonverbal expressions of pain except:
(A) A patient paces the floor.
(B) A patient wrings her hands.
(C) A patient resists care.
(D) A patient complains of sleepiness.

(21) When should a nurse aide use a transfer belt on a patient?
(A) When the patient is sleeping.
(B) During patient transfers and ambulation.
(C) Only when the patient requests it.
(D) For taking blood pressure measurements.

(22) A patient with severe depression should be assessed for the risk of:
(A) Suicidal ideation.
(B) Anger.
(C) Sadness.
(D) Elation.

(23) What is not a component of the MyPlate diet plan?
(A) Fruits.
(B) Vegetables.
(C) Grains.
(D) Water.

(24) You have made preparations to serve food to a patient in isolation. What is the most appropriate action before you enter the isolation room?
(A) Use PPE.
(B) Perform hand hygiene.
(C) Use a cotton nose mask.
(D) Use hand sanitizer.

(25) Which of the following can cause urinary incontinence?
(A) Gastroenteritis.
(B) Malaria.
(C) Spinal cord injury.
(D) Sepsis.

(26) Which of the following health promotion actions is important in patients with a colostomy?
(A) Colostomy training.
(B) Colostomy removal.
(C) Colostomy breakdown.
(D) Colostomy washing.

(27) When is it appropriate for a nurse aide to leave a patient's bed in a high position?
(A) When the patient is unattended.
(B) During meal times.
(C) While providing bedside care or treatment.
(D) After the patient has gone to sleep.

(28) A CNA bathes the whole body of a dependent patient while the patient lies in bed. This type of bath is known as a:

(A) Complete bed bath.

(B) Self-help bath.

(C) Partial bath.

(D) Full bath.

(29) What is not a common cause of visual impairment in the elderly?

(A) Cataracts.

(B) Glaucoma.

(C) Conjunctivitis.

(D) Macular degeneration.

(30) Which of the following steps is not correct when you want to communicate with a patient with dementia?

(A) Make eye contact.

(B) Respect the person's personal space.

(C) Never rush the person.

(D) Use distractions to facilitate communication.

(31) What is the purpose of a signaling device for a patient?

(A) To allow patients to listen to music.

(B) To enable patients to call for assistance.

(C) To monitor a patient's vital signs.

(D) To provide entertainment for patients.

(32) A 70-year-old woman sustains a hip fracture. The fracture is stabilized, and the patient is admitted to the orthopedic ward for postoperative care. Which of the following complications can result from this type of fracture?

(A) Hip tingling.

(B) Chronic hip pain.

(C) Weight loss.

(D) Fever.

(33) Which of the following measures can provide relief for patients with acute decompensation of chronic heart failure?
(A) Placement in the lithotomy position.
(B) Placement in the left lateral position.
(C) Placement in the Fowler's position.
(D) Lie down with the leg raised.

(34) Hypoglycemia can occur in a diabetic patient on insulin if the patient:
(A) Eats too much.
(B) Does not drink water.
(C) Misses a meal.
(D) Does not take his medications.

(35) A 30-year-old patient is brought to the emergency department due to difficulty breathing. He is diagnosed with influenza. Which of the following is the appropriate action to take on the patient?
(A) Isolate him.
(B) Care for him in the open ward.
(C) Discharge him.
(D) Provide outpatient care.

(36) An 82-year-old woman is brought to a nursing facility by her son. The CNA notices that the woman prefers to take brief walks to reflect and listen to music during midday meal hours. Which of the following is appropriate for the CNA to do?
(A) Ignore the situation.
(B) Do not allow the client to walk around at meal hours.
(C) Allow the client to walk short distances during the day and encourage her to eat whenever she returns.
(D) Report the situation to other family members.

(37) Which of the following is not a level in Maslow's Hierarchy of Needs?
(A) Safety and security needs.
(B) Physiological needs.
(C) Financial needs.
(D) Self-esteem needs.

(38) Which of the following is not one of the cognitive changes that can be associated with aging?
(A) Forgetfulness.
(B) Good hygiene and grooming.
(C) Depression.
(D) Disorientation.

(39) How should a nurse aide assist a patient with myopia in a healthcare setting?
(A) Ensure the patient has access to their prescribed eyeglasses.
(B) Administer eye drops regularly.
(C) Encourage the patient to focus on distant objects.
(D) Apply warm compresses to the eyes daily.

(40) Which of the following is not a hazard that a CNA will most likely encounter in a healthcare facility?
(A) Hospital-acquired infection.
(B) Exposure to chemicals.
(C) Radiation.
(D) Sunburn.

(41) One way a CNA can help to prevent the spread of infections is to:
(A) Clean up spills in a timely fashion.
(B) Set up equipment on time.
(C) Observe mealtimes.
(D) All of the above.

(42) When skin tears occur, what happens?
(A) The skin is dissected.
(B) Skin layers are peeled.
(C) The limb is amputated eventually.
(D) The skin flap always rejoins the skin on its own.

(43) What is a major concern in a patient who has just been diagnosed with Parkinson's?

(A) Memory loss.

(B) Vision loss.

(C) Falls.

(D Pain management.

(44) What does the term "abduction" refer to in the context of patient care and mobility?

(A) Removing harmful substances from the patient's room.

(B) The movement of a limb away from the midline of the body.

(C) Taking a patient away from their room for tests.

(D) Decreasing a patient's level of physical activity.

(45) You observe that a patient being managed for a cardiovascular condition is unable to breathe well when flat on her back in bed. What can you do?

(A) Recline the bed further.

(B) Make the bed rise slowly.

(C) Adjust the bed to a position of 120 degrees and observe.

(D) Adjust the bed to a position of 45 to 60 degrees and observe.

(46) Which of the following would you do first when you observe a patient who is restless?

(A) Use sedatives.

(B) Use antipsychotics.

(C) Calmly ask the patient what the problem is.

(D) Encourage the patient to exercise.

(47) Which of the following is not a safety device?

(A) Emergency alerts.

(B) Wander guards.

(C) Bedrails.

(D) Bodyguard.

(48) Why should a CNA stand on the weaker side of a patient who needs assistance with ambulation?

(A) To prevent falls.

(B) To build up the patient's weaker muscles.

(C) To increase the patient's grip.

(D) All of the above.

(49) What system is involved in the provision of support, mobility, and protection of vital organs?

(A) The circulatory system.

(B) The muscular system.

(C) The respiratory system.

(D) The musculoskeletal system.

(50) An 80-year-old woman has difficulty when she tries to move her knee joints. What disease is most likely responsible for this symptom?

(A) Rheumatic heart disease.

(B) Osteoarthritis.

(C) Slipped disc.

(D) Tuberculosis.

(51) Where are the blood cells produced?

(A) In the brain.

(B) In the bloodstream.

(C) In the bone marrow.

(D) All of the above.

(52) A two-year-old aspirated a cork. Which bronchus is the cork more likely to lodge in?

(A) Right bronchus.

(B) Left bronchus.

(C) Either bronchus.

(D) All of the above.

(53) A patient does not drink enough water or other fluids. This could cause:
(A) Constipation.
(B) Indigestion.
(C) Gastric cancer.
(D) All of the above.

(54) How many meninges enclose the brain?
(A) 1.
(B) 2.
(C) 3.
(D) 4.

(55) A 75-year-old man has Parkinson's disease. What are the most important things a CNA should do with this patient?
(A) Help with breathing.
(B) Provide warmth.
(C) Assist the patient to eat if tremors occur.
(D) All of the above.

(56) Which of the following must not be done during handwashing before CNA Jenny begins to feed a patient?
(A) Introduce herself appropriately.
(B) Apply soap to her hands.
(C) Moisten her hands and wrists.
(D) Touch the inside of the sink.

(57) A CNA dries his hands after he washes them. Where should he then place the used towels?
(A) On a hanger.
(B) In the trash can.
(C) By the bedside.
(D) All of the above.

(58) Which of the following can be used to turn off the faucet after handwashing?
(A) Hands.
(B) Feet.
(C) Clean paper towel.
(D) B and C.

(59) What is the first thing to do when a CNA wants to apply knee-high elastic stockings on a patient?
(A) Screen the patient.
(B) Turn the stockings inside out.
(C) Get a signaling device.
(D) Explain the procedure to the client.

(60) What position is the client in when knee-high stockings are applied?
(A) Prone.
(B) Supine.
(C) Seated.
(D) Standing.

(61) When measuring blood pressure, what is the correct position for the patient's arm?
(A) Hanging down at the side of the body.
(B) Raised above the head.
(C) At the same level as the heart.
(D) Crossed over the chest.

(62) What kind of footwear should a patient wear before he ambulates with a transfer belt?
(A) Bathroom slippers.
(B) Sneakers.
(C) Skates.
(D) Nonskid wear.

(63) What information must be discussed with a patient before ambulation?
(A) Movement pattern.
(B) Gait disorders.
(C) Vertebral column.
(D) Prearranged signal.

(64) How can a nursing assistant positively influence a patient's self-esteem?
(A) By discussing the patient's medical issues with other patients.
(B) Encouraging independence in daily activities as much as possible.
(C) Ignoring the patient's personal preferences.
(D) Limiting social interactions with the patient.

(65) Where should the bedpan be placed when a client wants to use it?
(A) Beside the client.
(B) Behind the client.
(C) Under the client.
(D) All of the above.

(66) Which of the following is not needed when a client needs to use a bedpan?
(A) Handwipes.
(B) Clean gloves.
(C) Signaling device.
(D) Transfer belt.

(67) Which practice is most effective in preventing the transmission of bloodborne pathogens?
(A) Engaging in regular exercise.
(B) Using PPE when handling blood or bodily fluids.
(C) Increasing the room temperature.
(D) Encouraging patients to eat a balanced diet.

(68) What should a CNA not do when a patient's dentures are cleaned?
(A) Wear clean gloves.
(B) Rinse the dentures in hot running water.
(C) Rinse the denture cup and lid.
(D) All of the above.

(69) Which of the following is not a part of dentures?
(A) Flange.
(B) Teeth.
(C) Base.
(D) Anchor.

(70) After a CNA cleans a patient's dentures, he must rinse the:

(A) Denture cup.

(B) Toothbrush.

(C) Toothpaste.

(D) A and B.

Test 1: Answers and Explanations

(1) (D) Delegate duties to other CNAs.

CNAs are certified health personnel whose responsibility is to assist patients with activities of daily living. They also perform other duties delegated to them by registered nurses. It is, however, not the duty of a CNA to delegate duties to other CNAs.

(2) (C) Acute care setting.

The acute care setting is where sudden emergency cases are managed. In the acute care setting, cases such as acute asthma, acute exacerbation of COPD, and acute pulmonary embolism are treated.

(3) (B) A CNA keeps the door open and discusses matters with a patient in a loud voice.

The goal of medical communication is to convey the message in clear terms but still ensure the patient's privacy and confidentiality. A CNA who keeps the door open and discusses matters with the patient in a loud voice may reveal confidential information to others.

(4) (A) Sit directly in front of the patient to talk.

Some patients who are hard of hearing learn to read lips. Therefore, it is recommended that healthcare workers position themselves directly in front of hard-of-hearing patients to make communication easier.

(5) (A) Measles.

Measles is an airborne infection transmitted through the respiratory tract. It presents with cough, nasal discharge, red eyes, and characteristic skin lesions. Patients with measles should be placed in respiratory isolation to prevent the spread of the disease.

(6) (B) Heart failure.

Heart failure is defined as the inability of the heart to pump enough blood to meet the metabolic demands of the body. This condition is characterized by classic symptoms such as dyspnea, orthopnea, swollen legs, and distended neck veins.

(7) (A) Fast and thready pulse.

Shock is a clinical state characterized by the failure of the heart to pump sufficient blood to meet the metabolic requirements of the body, which can result in cellular hypoxia. It is characterized by low blood pressure, a fast and thready pulse, cold and clammy extremities, and other features that depend on the cause of the shock.

(8) (D) Weight and height.

The BMI is used to classify individuals into normal weight, underweight, overweight, obese, and morbidly obese. The BMI of a patient correlates with cardiometabolic status. BMI is calculated with the formula BMI = weight in kg/square of the height in meters.

(9) (D) Fecal impaction.

Fecal impaction refers to hardened stools in the rectum or large bowel. The hardened stool becomes difficult to pass and may cause an obstruction. Forceful passage of the hard stools may cause anal tears.

(10) (A) Loss of bone tissue.

Osteoporosis is a condition characterized by soft bone due to demineralization of the bone, which becomes weak and brittle and prone to fracture. Osteoporosis can be caused by prolonged use of steroids, menopause and aging, and other disease conditions that cause bone demineralization.

(11) (B) Normal aging.

As people age, changes occur that affect how the body functions. Examples of normal forgetfulness are misplacement of commonly used items, such as keys or eyeglasses, or having a word on the tip of the tongue and being unable to say it.

(12) (C) To elevate the patient's feet higher than the head.

In the Trendelenburg position, the patient is placed on their back and the lower body is elevated higher than the head. This position is used to improve blood circulation to the brain, particularly in cases of shock or low blood pressure. It allows gravity to assist in increasing the blood flow to the brain and vital organs.

(13) (C) Cataract.

Cataracts are common among elderly patients. They arise from the opacification of the lens of the eyes. Risk factors include age, chronic steroid use, diabetes, etc. The visual loss created by cataracts is reversible with cataract surgery.

(14) (A) Passes watery stool three or more times in a day.

Diarrhea occurs when a patient passes loose, watery stools three or more times a day. Loose stool is any stool that takes the shape of the container. Diarrhea signifies a gastrointestinal problem such as gastroenteritis. Management is to treat the cause and replace lost fluids.

(15) (A) Long-term oxygen therapy.

Long-term oxygen therapy may be required in COPD patients. For patients who meet the criteria, long-term oxygen therapy helps to prolong life and reduce mortality.

Although patients with COPD may have a cough, treatment of the underlying exacerbation rather than cough medication is usually the standard.

(16) (B) To check for the immediate blood sugar levels at any time.

A random blood sugar test is conducted to measure the amount of glucose in the patient's blood at the time of the test, without regard to the time since the patient's last meal.

(17) (C) Eyes.

When a patient's hair is washed, the eyes should be protected by a cloth to prevent irritation and redness.

(18) (C) Parenteral feeding.

Parenteral feeding is the best form of feeding from the options listed. The patient with a bowel obstruction requires nutrient delivery that bypasses the bowels. This will ensure bowel rest as well as adequate evaluation and treatment of the bowel disease. Neither nasogastric feeding nor oral feeding provides bowel rest.

(19) (A) Carbohydrates.

Glucose is one of the simple sugars that form the building blocks of carbohydrates. It is a six-carbon sugar that is essential for most of the body's biochemical activities. Glucose can be generated from amino acids and other substrates through a process called gluconeogenesis.

(20) (D) A patient complains of sleepiness.

Sleepiness is not a nonverbal expression of pain. Nonverbal expressions include restlessness, pacing, rocking, and refusal of care. CNAs need to be observant of these signs and report them to the nurse when observed.

(21) (B) During patient transfers and ambulation.

A transfer belt is also known as a gait belt. It is used to assist patients who are partially mobile and need help moving from one place to another, such as from a bed to a wheelchair. The belt provides a secure way to support the patient and reduces the risk of falls or injuries during these movements.

(22) (A) Suicidal ideation.

Patients with severe depression are at high risk of suicide or deliberate self-harm.

(23) (D) Water.

The MyPlate diet plan includes the recommended proportions of fruits, grains, proteins, vegetables, and dairy in meals. Water is not part of the MyPlate diet plan.

(24) (A) Use PPE.

The use of PPE is very important when a CNA serves food to patients in isolation. Although hand hygiene is very important, the only specific protective action in this scenario is the use of PPE to prevent the transmission of communicable diseases.

(25) (C) Spinal cord injury.

A spinal cord injury, such as a partial or total transection of the spinal cord, can result in symptoms such as urinary retention or urinary incontinence. Nerve signals from the spinal cord control the micturition reflex. Damage to the fibers of the spinal cord that supply the pelvis may affect the control of urination.

(26) (A) Colostomy training.

Colostomy training involves training the colostomy to achieve an elimination pattern just like the bowel and bladder. Colostomy breakdown, training, and washing are not health promotion services.

(27) (C) While providing bedside care or treatment.

The high position of a bed is used to bring the patient up to a level that is easier for the caregiver to access without straining their back. This position is especially useful when performing tasks like changing dressings, conducting examinations, or assisting with personal hygiene. It is important to lower the bed to its lowest position when the task is completed, particularly when the patient is sleeping or unattended, to reduce the risk of falls.

(28) (A) Complete bed bath.

A complete bed bath is recommended for a patient who is completely immobilized. The patient's whole body is cleaned and bathed.

(29) (C) Conjunctivitis.

Although conjunctivitis can cause eye pain, itching, and diplopia, it is not a common cause of blindness at any age. Conjunctivitis can be classified as infective or non-infective. Infective conjunctivitis commonly occurs due to viral and bacterial causes.

(30) (D) Use distractions to facilitate communication.

With patients with cognitive impairment like dementia, extra efforts should be made to make sure the message is conveyed as simply as possible. The speaker should maintain eye contact, respect the patient's personal space, and never rush the patient. Distractions do not facilitate communication.

(31) (B) To enable patients to call for assistance.

A signaling device like a call bell or button is a tool provided to patients that enables them to alert the nursing staff or caregivers when they need help. This can be vital for patients who may require immediate assistance, have a medical emergency, need help with basic needs like using the restroom, or have other care requirements.

(32) (B) Chronic hip pain.

Patients with hip fractures are at risk of avascular necrosis of the femur. This condition presents with chronic pain in the hip joints. The patient may also walk with an antalgic gait. Sickle cell disease patients are also at risk of developing avascular necrosis of the femur head.

(33) (C) Placement in the Fowler's position.

A patient with acute decompensation of chronic heart failure will most likely present with pulmonary edema, which involves fluids in the lung parenchyma. This leads to coughing, difficulty breathing, and fast breathing. Placement in the Fowler's position relieves the symptoms somewhat.

(34) (C) Misses a meal.

Hypoglycemia is a reduction in the serum sugar below 3.0 mmol/l. It causes headaches, sweating, weakness, and, in severe cases, fainting. Hypoglycemia in diabetic patients is most commonly from overdose of medications or missed meals.

(35) (A) Isolate him.

Patients with diagnosed or suspected influenza should be placed in respiratory isolation to prevent the spread of the disease. Tuberculosis is also managed this way.

(36) (C) Allow the client to walk short distances during the day and encourage her to eat whenever she returns.

To force decisions on patients is prohibited as they have the right to make choices and exercise control over their lives. Though the client's desired activity time is during midday meal hours, the CNA should practice the principle of autonomy. The patient should be allowed to go on brief walks for short distances during the day and encouraged to eat whenever she returns.

(37) (C) Financial needs.

Financial need is not a level in Maslow's Hierarchy of Needs. The different levels include safety and security, love and belonging, self-esteem, and self-actualization.

(38) (B) Good hygiene and grooming.

Cognitive abilities begin to decline as a person ages. This might be linked to certain neurological disorders such as dementia, delirium, etc. Cognitive changes in the aged include forgetfulness, poor hygiene and grooming, depression, disorientation, memory loss, and poor concentration.

(39) (A) Ensure the patient has access to their prescribed eyeglasses.

Myopia is commonly known as nearsightedness, and it is a vision condition where a person sees close objects clearly but struggles to see objects that are far away. For a patient with myopia, it is important to ensure that they have easy access to their prescribed eyeglasses, as these are essential for them to see clearly at a distance.

(40) (D) Sunburn.

CNAs are unlikely to experience sunburns in a healthcare facility. They are more likely to be exposed to hospital-acquired infections, exposure to chemicals, or radiation due to the nature of their work.

(41) (A) Clean up spills in a timely fashion.

A CNA should quickly clean up spills to maintain sanitary conditions and prevent slips and falls.

(42) (B) Skin layers are peeled.

Skin tears occur when there is a break that has peeled layers of the skin. The skin layer can be partially removed or totally lifted. The skin flap does not always rejoin the rest of the skin on its own.

(43) (C) Falls.

Parkinson's affects the basal ganglia, which plays a critical role in balance. So, patients just diagnosed with Parkinson's might easily lose their balance. They might also have stiff muscles and have poor mobility, which can lead to falls.

(44) (B) The movement of a limb away from the midline of the body.

"Abduction" refers to the movement of a limb or other part away from the midline of the body, or from another part. This is a term that nurse aides need to be familiar with, especially when assisting with exercises or movements prescribed in a patient's care plan.

(45) (D) Adjust the bed to a position of 45 to 60 degrees and observe.

When the bed is adjusted to a position of 45 to 60 degrees, the fluid in the lungs will move downward and allow the patient to breathe.

(46) (C) Calmly ask the patient what the problem is.

When encountering a patient who is restless, the first and most important step is to communicate directly with the patient to understand the root cause of their restlessness.

By calmly asking the patient about the problem, you can gain valuable information about their current state, needs, or discomforts. This approach is non-invasive and prioritizes patient-centered care.

(47) (D) Bodyguard.

A bodyguard, in the context of healthcare and patient safety, is not considered a safety device. Safety devices in healthcare settings are typically tools or systems designed to protect patients from harm or assist in their care. Emergency alerts, wander guards, and bedrails are all examples of such devices.

(48) (A) To prevent falls.

A CNA should stand on the weaker side of a patient who needs assistance with ambulation primarily to prevent falls. When a patient has a weaker side, they are more prone to losing balance or falling towards that side. By positioning themselves on the weaker side, the CNA can provide better support and stabilization for the patient, and reduce the risk of falls.

(49) (D) The musculoskeletal system.

The musculoskeletal system provides structural support, protects vital organs, and facilitates movement. The muscular system alone is not able to provide adequate structural support. The circulatory system is involved in the transportation of blood and nutrients around the body. The respiratory system is involved in the exchange of gases.

(50) (B) Osteoarthritis.

In osteoarthritis, the cartilage that protects the bone ends during movement begins to wear out. When the bones move, they rub directly on each other, which results in pain, discomfort, and sometimes, swelling.

(51) (C) In the bone marrow.

Blood cells are produced in the bone marrow. This includes red blood cells, white blood cells, and platelets.

(52) (A) Right bronchus.

The right bronchus is wider than the left bronchus. It also enters the lungs at a lesser angle, which makes it straighter than the left. This increases the risk of aspiration in the right bronchus.

(53) (A) Constipation.

Inadequate water or fluid intake can cause constipation. Water is essential for digestion as it helps to soften stools and maintain regular bowel movements. When the body is dehydrated, the colon absorbs more water from the food waste, which can make the stool hard and difficult to pass.

(54) (C) 3.

The brain is enclosed by three layers of protective coverings called meninges. These three meninges are the dura mater, arachnoid mater, and pia mater. The dura mater is the outermost layer, tough and durable, providing the primary protective barrier. The arachnoid mater is the middle layer, which is a web-like structure filled with cerebrospinal fluid that cushions the brain. The pia mater is the innermost layer, which is a thin, delicate membrane that closely adheres to the surface of the brain.

(55) (C) Assist the patient to eat if tremors occur.

A patient with Parkinson's probably will experience a lot of tremors that might make eating very difficult, so assistance is required.

(56) (D) Touch the inside of the sink.

When they wash their hands, CNAs should not touch the inside of the sink, which may contain bacteria and other contaminants.

(57) (B) In the trash can.

The paper towels should be disposed of in the trash can or other appropriate waste containers after use. They should not be reused.

(58) (C) Clean paper towel.

After handwashing, it is recommended to use a clean paper towel to turn off the faucet. This practice is advised to prevent recontamination of the hands. When hands are washed, they are cleaned of germs and contaminants. However, the faucet handles may still be contaminated because they were touched before handwashing.

(59) (D) Explain the procedure to the client.

The first step a CNA should take when planning to apply knee-high elastic stockings to a patient is to explain the procedure to the client. This is an essential part of patient care, as it ensures that the patient is informed and comfortable with the procedure. Clear communication helps to alleviate any anxiety or confusion the patient might have and allows them to give informed consent.

(60) (B) Supine.

When applying knee-high stockings to a client, the client should be in the supine position. The supine position means lying on the back, face upwards. This position is ideal for applying such stockings because it allows for easy access to the legs and ensures that the stockings can be applied smoothly and evenly without causing discomfort to the client. It also helps to ensure that the stockings are not twisted or unevenly distributed, which can happen if the client is in a seated or standing position.

(61) (C) At the same level as the heart.

When you measure a patient's blood pressure, it is important to position the patient's arm so that it is at heart level. This position ensures the most accurate reading. If the arm is too high or too low relative to the heart, it can affect the blood pressure reading and potentially result in an inaccurate assessment. The arm should be supported and relaxed, neither hanging down nor raised above the head, nor crossed over the chest.

(62) (D) Nonskid wear.

Patients should put on nonskid shoes before they ambulate with a transfer belt to reduce the risk of slips and falls.

(63) (A) Movement pattern.

Before ambulating a patient, it is important to discuss the movement pattern with them. This includes explaining how they will be moved, the steps involved in the process, and what is expected of them during ambulation. Discussing the movement pattern helps prepare the patient for the activity, ensures they understand their role in the process, and can reduce anxiety or confusion. It also helps to ensure the safety and efficiency of the ambulation process.

(64) (B) Encouraging independence in daily activities as much as possible.

Promoting a patient's independence in daily activities is a key way to boost their self-esteem. When patients are encouraged and supported to do as much for themselves as they can safely manage, it helps them feel more capable and confident.

(65) (C) Under the client.

When a client needs to use a bedpan, it should be placed under the client. This positioning is essential for the practical and effective use of the bedpan. Placing the bedpan under the client ensures that it is in the correct position to collect waste.

(66) (D) Transfer belt.

When a client needs to use a bedpan, a transfer belt is not usually needed. The main use of a transfer belt is to assist patients who are mobile enough to stand or walk with support, especially during transfers and ambulation. In the case of a bedpan, the client is usually in bed and does not need to be mobilized to use the bedpan.

(67) (B) Using PPE when handling blood or bodily fluids.

Personal protective equipment, such as gloves, gowns, masks, and eye protection, is essential in preventing the transmission of bloodborne pathogens. This equipment creates a barrier between the healthcare worker and potentially infectious materials, and reduces the risk of exposure to bloodborne pathogens like HIV, Hepatitis B, and Hepatitis C.

(68) (B) Rinse the dentures in hot running water.

When a CNA cleans a patient's dentures, they should not rinse the dentures in hot running water. This is because hot water can warp or damage the dentures. It can alter their fit and make them uncomfortable or unusable for the patient. Dentures are made from materials that can be sensitive to extreme temperatures, so it's important to use lukewarm or cold water for rinsing.

(69) (D) Anchor.

In dentures, an 'anchor' is not a part. Dentures consist of three main components: the base, the teeth, and the flange. The base of the denture is designed to sit on the gums and is usually made from a gum-colored acrylic material. The teeth are attached to this base and are made from either porcelain or acrylic. The flange is the part of the denture that extends into the vestibule (the area between the lips, cheeks, and gums) and helps to provide support and stability to the denture.

(70) (D) A and B.

CNAs should always rinse the denture cup and toothbrush after the dentures are cleaned. The toothbrush should then be returned to the designated toothbrush container.

Test 2: Questions

(1) What is not a requirement for a health worker to qualify as a certified CNA?

(A) Valid CNA certification.

(B) Ability to lift, push, and pull objects of at least 30 pounds.

(C) Basic computer skills.

(D) Advanced cardiac life support certification.

(2) A 35-year-old man comes to the ER with an insidious-onset cough, difficulty with breathing, and a fever. He is admitted to the medical ward. Which of the following words most correctly describes this patient?

(A) Outpatient.

(B) Inpatient.

(C) Emergency.

(D) Urgency.

(3) As a CNA, how can you help meet your patients' physical needs?

(A) Help them attend a musical concert.

(B) Help them eat.

(C) Help them with sexual satisfaction.

(D) Help them attain spiritual growth.

(4) What is the right communication approach when CNA Miguel visits the room of a patient with a visual impairment?

(A) He should knock and introduce himself.

(B) He should stand in front of the patient when he talks.

(C) He should not introduce himself, so as not to startle the patient.

(D) He should not knock on the door.

(5) A 10-year-old boy is brought to the ER with complaints of rice-water stool for the past three days. Stool microscopy, culture, and sensitivity confirm the diagnosis of cholera. Which precautions should be employed with this patient?

(A) Droplet precautions.

(B) Airborne precautions.

(C) Contact precautions.

(D) No precautions.

(6) A 35-year-old man is admitted to the medical ward for community-acquired pneumonia. Which vital signs measurement is most important in this patient?

(A) Pulse rate.

(B) Respiratory rate.

(C) Body mass index.

(D) Heart rate.

(7) At which of the following anatomical locations can the radial pulse be measured?

(A) The wrist.

(B) The foot.

(C) The elbow.

(D) The armpit.

(8) Which approach can be used to feed patients who cannot tolerate food orally?

(A) Rectal approach.

(B) Gastrostomy tube approach.

(C) Intranasal approach.

(D) A and B.

(9) Incontinence is a term used to describe the:

(A) Inability to pass urine.

(B) Inability to pass stool.

(C) Inability to control vomiting.

(D) Inability to control the release of stool and urine.

(10) A patient with arthritis should be encouraged to:

(A) Avoid movement.

(B) Avoid painkillers.

(C) Do minimal exercise.

(D) Nothing.

(11) Mr. Gold comes to the hospital to seek medical care. He was recently diagnosed with dementia. How should a CNA not approach this patient?

(A) Take a clinical approach first.

(B) Eliminate distractions.

(C) Make eye contact, preferably at eye level.

(D) Observe the patient's body language.

(12) What should a CNA not do to promote the physical comfort of a dying person?
(A) Reposition the patient per the care plan.
(B) Provide frequent skin care.
(C) Provide frequent mouth care.
(D) Manage all comfort care needs.

(13) What is the definitive treatment for cataracts?
(A) Surgery.
(B) Glasses.
(C) Drugs.
(D) Observation.

(14) A 70-year-old stroke survivor complains of difficulty moving her bowels. She has not had a bowel movement in four days except for a hard stool pellet. Rectal examination reveals hard stools. What is the most likely diagnosis?
(A) Fecal impaction.
(B) Anal fissure.
(C) Anal fistula.
(D) Anal abscess.

(15) A 55-year-old farmer with a significant history of smoking, alcohol, multiple sexual partners, and hypertension develops a cough productive of sputum for four months. He is diagnosed with lung cancer. Which of the following is the most significant risk factor for his condition?
(A) Alcohol.
(B) Hypertension.
(C) Multiple sexual partners.
(D) Smoking.

(16) A 56-year-old man is scheduled to be moved to the operating room for an elective procedure. The CNA arrives to move the patient. Which of the following should the CNA do?
(A) Move the patient with the assumption that he knows where he is being moved.
(B) Tell the patient how he can help to make the transfer easier.
(C) Rush the patient.
(D) Allow the patient to put his arms around the CNA's neck for support.

(17) A 65-year-old woman with multiple sclerosis must be assisted with a shower because she is unstable and has a history of previous falls. Which of the following is most appropriate for the patient?
(A) She should stand while she showers.
(B) She should use a shower stool.
(C) She should have a bed bath.
(D) She should lie supine while she showers.

(18) What is a symptom of lactose intolerance?
(A) Constipation.
(B) Vomiting blood.
(C) Bloating.
(D) Chest pain.

(19) What kind of food are amino acids?
(A) Protein.
(B) Fats.
(C) Oils.
(D) Carbohydrate.

(20) Mrs. Murphy is a 52-year-old woman who has had hip pain for the past two months. She decides to wait five more months before surgery. All of the following could contribute to her pain tolerance except:
(A) Her family and culture.
(B) Her past experiences with pain.
(C) The pleasure she gains from pain.
(D) Her emotional state.

(21) Mr. Williams, a 66-year-old man, is in the terminal stage of liver cancer. He requests that a clergyman perform some rituals before his death. What is the appropriate thing to do?
(A) Ignore his wishes.
(B) Explain that the rituals will not prevent his death.
(C) Report his request to a nurse.
(D) Seek the consent of his family members.

(22) A 68-year-old patient develops an insidious onset of irrational behavior on the ward. She is diagnosed with delirium. Part of the management goals for the patient should be to:

(A) Reorient the patient to time, place, or person.

(B) Sedate the patient.

(C) Give the patient antibiotics.

(D) Give the patient analgesics.

(23) A 34-year-old woman with obesity and diet-controlled diabetes mellitus comes to the clinic to see the dietician. What is the unit of measurement for the amount of energy present in food?

(A) Joules.

(B) Power.

(C) Calories.

(D) Volts.

(24) Which of the following patients would most likely struggle to swallow food?

(A) Diabetic patient.

(B) Stroke survivor.

(C) Hypertensive.

(D) Patient with a Hepatitis B infection.

(25) Mr. Jack, a 55-year-old patient, develops an insidious onset of urinary incontinence. Which nonpharmacological measures can be beneficial for him?

(A) Bowel training.

(B) Bladder training.

(C) Intravenous fluids.

(D) Regular exercise.

(26) A 68-year-old patient with Alzheimer's disease undergoes a procedure where fluid is passed through her anus to remove feces. What is this procedure called?

(A) Fecal disimpaction.

(B) Elimination.

(C) Enema.

(D) Bowel lavage.

(27) Which of the following is a protein-rich food?
(A) Orange.
(B) Beans.
(C) Yam.
(D) Potatoes.

(28) A patient is helped to clean body parts that may cause odor. What is this called?
(A) Full bath.
(B) Partial bed bath.
(C) Self-help cleaning.
(D) Cleaning up.

(29) Fecal impaction can be treated with:
(A) Digital dis-impaction.
(B) Gastric lavage.
(C) Rectal manometry.
(D) Intravenous fluids.

(30) Which of the following is not a type of dementia?
(A) Alzheimer's dementia.
(B) Lewy-body dementia.
(C) Vascular dementia.
(D) Amnestic dementia.

(31) Which mobility assistance device provides a place for the CNA to put their hands?
(A) Shoulder grip.
(B) Hand belt.
(C) Gait belt.
(D) Cane.

(32) Which of the following is not recommended care for a patient on oxygen therapy?
(A) Check regularly to ensure the tubes are not kinked.
(B) Inform the nurse about changes in flow rate.
(C) Provide good skin care around the cannula.
(D) Remove the cannula to perform facial care.

(33) A 46-year-old multiple sclerosis patient develops progressive difficulty with swallowing due to problems with throat muscle coordination. The patient is at risk of:
(A) Aspiration pneumonia.
(B) Hospital-acquired pneumonia.
(C) Interstitial pneumonia.
(D) Atypical pneumonia.

(34) Hyperglycemia can occur in a diabetic patient on insulin therapy if the patient:
(A) Misses his medication.
(B) Eats too little.
(C) Exercises.
(D) Drinks too much water.

(35) Which of the following is not a reason for indwelling catheter use?
(A) Surgery.
(B) Postoperative use.
(C) To relieve urinary obstruction.
(D) To treat urinary tract infections.

(36) Which of the following is appropriate for a woman who has a hard time coping with losses and adjustment?
(A) Inform other patients about the woman's worries.
(B) Validate the woman's concerns and express empathy.
(C) Ignore the woman's concerns.
(D) Tell the woman her worries are foolish.

(37) A CNA meets a 25-year-old client who is currently homeless and does not have access to food, water, or shelter. Which level of Maslow's Hierarchy of Needs is most relevant to this client?
(A) Financial needs.
(B) Self-esteem needs.
(C) Physiological needs.
(D) Self-actualization needs.

(38) A 75-year-old man's wife complains that he has become forgetful in the past few months. He also has difficulty following conversations and completing tasks. What condition might the man have?

(A) Alzheimer's disease.

(B) Vascular dementia.

(C) Lewy-body dementia.

(D) Parkinson's disease.

(39) The elderly should not be encouraged to:

(A) Participate in rcligious activities based on beliefs.

(B) Exercise.

(C) Interact with friends and family members.

(D) Stay silent, as people may not understand their speech patterns.

(40) How should a nursing assistant respond when a patient is in denial about their medical condition?

(A) Confront the patient aggressively about the reality of their condition.

(B) Ignore the patient's feelings and proceed with the care plan.

(C) Provide support and gently encourage communication about their condition.

(D) Tell the patient that denial will worsen their condition.

(41) A CNA working in the radiological unit should:

(A) Do regular checks of exposure level.

(B) Limit exposure.

(C) Always wear PPE.

(D) All of the above.

(42) One major risk factor for skin tears in the elderly is:

(A) Aging.

(B) Heart failure.

(C) Falls.

(D) All of the above.

(43) What is one strategy to prevent falls among people with neurological impairments?
(A) Always remain with such patients when they use the restroom.
(B) Help such patients with personal hygiene activities.
(C) Perform regular observation.
(D) All of the above.

(44) What is not one of the major risks associated with falls in elderly people?
(A) Hemorrhage.
(B) Fractures.
(C) Hematoma.
(D) Allergies.

(45) When a patient with a high risk of falls arrives on the ward, a CNA should:
(A) Learn the patient's history.
(B) Categorize the patient as high risk for falls.
(C) Collaborate with other healthcare professionals.
(D) All of the above.

(46) A patient begins to speak loudly and move restlessly on his bed. The CNA switches on the TV to a program the patient enjoys. He calms down after that. What technique was displayed here?
(A) Distraction.
(B) Professional restraint.
(C) Round monitoring.
(D) Aggression burst.

(47) One advantage of entry supervision systems is that:
(A) They allow control of access.
(B) They prevent falls.
(C) They limit medication side effects.
(D) All of the above.

(48) What is one of the most overlooked places to contract diseases and/or come into contact with germs in a healthcare facility?

(A) Toilet seat.

(B) Handrails.

(C) Bed.

(D) Floor.

(49) Which of the following statements about the human skeletal system is wrong?

(A) There are 206 bones in the adult human body.

(B) The skeletal system is divided into the axial and appendicular skeletons.

(C) Joints are held together by tendons.

(D) Muscles have origins and insertions.

(50) A 27-year-old man is diagnosed with osteomalacia. What nutrient deficiency causes this condition?

(A) Calcium deficiency.

(B) Vitamin B deficiency.

(C) Vitamin D deficiency.

(D) Potassium deficiency.

(51) Which cells help defend the body?

(A) White blood cells.

(B) Red blood cells.

(C) Platelets.

(D) All of the above.

(52) What type of blood flows in the pulmonary vein?

(A) Oxygenated blood.

(B) Deoxygenated blood.

(C) Arthrombocytic blood.

(D) All of the above.

(53) A patient who suffers from diarrhea needs more:

(A) Food.

(B) Fluids.

(C) Proteins.

(D) Vitamins.

(54) What is the closest meningeal layer to the brain?
(A) The dura mater.
(B) The pia mater.
(C) The arachnoid mater.
(D) The subarachnoid mater.

(55) A 62-year-old woman is admitted to the ward with weakness on the right side of her body. She then regains all function. What is the most likely reason for what happened?
(A) TIA.
(B) Stroke.
(C) Pulmonary embolism.
(D) Acute encephalopathy.

(56) How should CNAs clean their fingernails when they wash their hands?
(A) Rub the fingernails against the palm of the same hand.
(B) Rub the fingernails against each other.
(C) Rub the fingernails against the palm.
(D) Rub the fingernails against the palm of the opposite hand.

(57) What is a simple solution for a patient who repeatedly returns to the clinic with diarrhea related to diet and hygiene?
(A) Handwashing.
(B) Antibiotics.
(C) Colonoscopy.
(D) All of the above.

(58) During handwashing, how should the hands be dried?
(A) Start from the wrists.
(B) Start from the palm.
(C) Start from the fingertips.
(D) Start from any point.

(59) What condition is most likely to require a knee-high stocking?
(A) Hypertension.
(B) Pulmonary edema.
(C) Varicose veins.
(D) All of the above.

(60) What body part should the foot of the stocking be placed over?
(A) Toes.
(B) Foot.
(C) Heel.
(D) All of the above.

(61) Where should a CNA place the transfer belt to move a patient effectively?
(A) At the hips.
(B) At the waist.
(C) At the back.
(D) At the legs.

(62) When should a transfer belt be removed?
(A) Before movement.
(B) After movement.
(C) During movement.
(D) Not until the patient is discharged.

(63) A CNA needs to move a patient from the bed to a chair. She should:
(A) Support the patient.
(B) Not pull the patient with the transfer belt.
(C) Use the transfer belt as a pulley alone.
(D) All of the above.

(64) During the 40th week of pregnancy, which of these would be a focus of care for a nurse aide?
(A) Encouraging the patient to start new intense exercise routines.
(B) Assisting with mobility and comfort due to increased body size.
(C) Introducing a drastically different diet.
(D) Recommending the patient to travel extensively.

(65) What should CNA Lee pay special attention to when a patient needs assistance with a bedpan?
(A) Color of gloves.
(B) Posture.
(C) Not to contaminate the bedpan.
(D) Not to contaminate himself when the gloves are removed.

(66) Which of the following does not provide sufficient privacy for a patient who needs to use a bedpan?
(A) A curtain.
(B) A screen.
(C) A door.
(D) Bedsheets

(67) In which of the following situations is it most appropriate to raise the head of the patient's bed?
(A) When the patient is experiencing difficulty breathing.
(B) When the patient is in a deep sleep.
(C) For all patients, regardless of their condition.
(D) When the patient has lower back pain.

(68) Why is accurate urine measurement important?
(A) To monitor a patient's hydration and kidney function.
(B) To check the patient's ability to follow instructions.
(C) To determine the patient's intelligence level.
(D) To assess the patient's mobility skills.

(69) What are the conditions that might require a patient to use dentures?
(A) Gum disease.
(B) Intraoral cancer.
(C) Injury.
(D) All of the above.

(70) When should dentures be rinsed?
(A) Before they are brushed with toothpaste.
(B) After they are brushed with toothpaste.
(C) After they are placed in the denture cup.
(D) A and B.

Test 2: Answers and Explanations

(1) (D) Advanced cardiac life support certification.

CNAs are not expected to have an advanced life support certificate. They are, however, required to have basic cardiopulmonary resuscitation skills. They are also expected to be physically fit enough to be able to assist in patient transfers and movements of objects.

(2) (B) Inpatient.

The term "inpatient" is used to describe patients admitted to a health facility. Although this patient was rushed to the emergency department, the term "emergency" is not the best word to describe him after his admission to the medical ward.

(3) (B) Help them eat.

One of the roles of CNAs is to help patients with activities of daily living. They also help patients meet social, physical, biological, and spiritual needs. Patients must eat, so a CNA can help with this.

(4) (A) He should knock and introduce himself.

A CNA should announce his arrival with a greeting when he visits the room of a patient with a visual impairment. This ensures that he does not startle the patient. It also helps the patient prepare mentally for the CNA's arrival and to know who they are talking to.

(5) (C) Contact precautions.

This patient needs to be placed on contact precaution measures. Anyone who comes in contact with this patient should wash their hands because cholera is transmitted via the fecal-oral route.

(6) (B) Respiratory rate.

Most patients with lung infections such as pneumonia have an increased respiratory rate. After treatment is initiated, the respiratory rate gradually returns to normal.

(7) (A) The wrist.

The wrist is the anatomical landmark used to check the radial pulse. The radial artery is the artery on the lateral side of the wrist. The ulnar artery is on the medial side of the wrist.

(8) (B) Gastrostomy tube approach.

Patients with a severe gastric outlet obstruction or other conditions that obstruct intestinal drainage cannot be fed orally. A gastrostomy tube is connected to the stomach so the patient can be fed through the tube.

(9) (D) Inability to control the release of stool and urine.

Incontinence is the inability to control the flow of feces and urine. It may be caused by a number of factors. The factors may be psychological, physical, and behavioral.

(10) (C) Do minimal exercise.

Arthritis is a condition characterized by inflammation of the joints. It can be osteoarthritis, rheumatoid arthritis, or septic arthritis. Other conditions that present with arthritis include gout, psoriasis, etc. Patients with this condition should do minimal exercise daily.

(11) (A) Take a clinical approach first.

In communication with persons with dementia, it is recommended that healthcare personnel are social before being clinical. This approach allows the person to feel comfortable before they are touched or otherwise interacted with medically.

(12) (D) Manage all comfort care needs.

It is recommended to report conditions such as pain, difficulty breathing, constipation, nausea, vomiting, or anxiety to the nurse so that measures can be taken to relieve these sources of discomfort.

(13) (A) Surgery.

The definitive treatment for cataracts is surgery. During the surgery, the crystalline lens of the eye is removed, and an artificial lens is implanted. The surgery fully corrects the visual loss. Patients with mild symptoms may benefit from conservative management rather than surgery.

(14) (A) Fecal impaction.

Fecal impaction is a complication of chronic constipation. In constipation, water is absorbed from the stool, and the resultant hard stool becomes difficult to pass. Fecal impaction can result in intestinal obstruction. Chronic straining may also cause anal tears and hemorrhoids.

(15) (D) Smoking.

Smoking is a strong risk factor for lung cancer. As for COPD, tobacco smoking significantly increases the lifetime risk of lung cancer. Screening for lung cancer is recommended for patients who have ever smoked. Smoking cessation is advised for all patients.

(16) (B) Tell the patient how he can help to make the transfer easier.

When a patient is to be transferred from one point to another within the healthcare facility, the patient should be first informed of the reason for the transfer. Then, the patient's mobility issues must be confirmed, and the patient should be given instructions on how to position his body to make the transfer easier.

(17) (B) She should use a shower stool.

The shower stool is equipment that is commonly found in assisted living facilities. It is recommended for use by patients who are unstable to shower while upright. Shower stools help to prevent falls.

(18) (C) Bloating.

Patients with lactose intolerance cannot digest lactose, a common sugar found in milk and other dairy products. Lactose intolerance presents with bloating, abdominal discomfort, indigestion, abdominal pain, etc. It does not present with constipation or vomiting of blood.

(19) (A) Protein.

Amino acids are the building blocks of proteins. Proteins are essential for building most of the cellular structures in the body. When proteins are digested, they release amino acids. The amino acids are then used for metabolic activities or converted to glucose for metabolic use.

(20) (C) The pleasure she gains from the pain.

An individual's family and culture, their past experiences with pain, and their emotional state are all factors that could influence response to pain, and, in this case, Mrs. Murphy's decision to wait five more months for the surgery.

(21) (C) Report his request to a nurse.

Certain rituals may need to be followed per a person's religious or cultural beliefs. Make sure that the necessary arrangements have been made to allow the rituals to be carried out according to the family's wishes. When a patient expresses such wishes, the request should be reported to the nurse.

(22) (A) Reorient the patient to time, place, and person.

Delirium is an acute confusional state that is characterized by disorganized behaviors, irrational speech, disorganized body movements, and disorientation to time, place, and person. Delirium is usually secondary to an underlying disease, which should be evaluated and treated.

(23) (C) Calories.

The amount of energy that a food provides is measured in calories. The number of calories supplied by a meal is important in the creation of dietary plans for patients being treated for diseases like diabetes and hypertension. Diets that are high in calories are discouraged in people with obesity, diabetes, and hypertension.

(24) (B) Stroke survivor.

Stroke survivors often have difficulty with swallowing. This is mostly because stroke causes weakness in muscles.

(25) (B) Bladder training.

Bladder training is a nonpharmacological measure that can be beneficial in patients with urinary incontinence. Urinary incontinence may arise from damage to the bladder neck or loss of nerve supply to the pelvis. It may also occur as overflow incontinence in patients with bladder outlet obstruction.

(26) (C) Enema.

An enema is a procedure done to remove impacted fecal matter from a patient's rectum. Fecal impaction most commonly follows chronic unrelieved constipation. The fecal matter becomes hard and pellet-like and is often difficult to pass. Manual disimpaction or enemas can be used to treat the condition.

(27) (B) Beans.

All the other classes of food listed are not as rich in protein as beans are. Other sources of protein include fish, eggs, meat, and meat products.

(28) (B) Partial bed bath.

A partial bed bath involves only specific body parts that are prone to odor, such as the skin folds, armpits, neck, and face.

(29) (A) Digital dis-impaction.

Fecal impaction occurs when hardened fecal matter obstructs the rectum. Intestinal obstruction from impaction may present with tenesmus, abdominal pain, and bloating. Digital dis-impaction is the treatment of choice.

(30) (D) Amnestic dementia.

Dementia is a chronic progressive degenerative disease that is associated with impairment in cognition, memory, and intellect. There are several forms of dementia. Alzheimer's dementia is the most common. Others are vascular, frontotemporal, and Lewy-body dementia.

(31) (C) Gait belt.

A gait belt is used to stabilize a patient during transfer. It is most advisable to hold the patient by the gait belt to prevent injuries and falls.

(32) (D) Remove the cannula to perform facial care.

When they provide facial care for patients on oxygen, CNAs should check regularly to ensure the tubes are not kinked. They should also inform the nurse about changes in flow rates and provide good skin care around the cannula. However, it is wrong to remove the cannula to perform facial care.

(33) (A) Aspiration pneumonia.

Patients with disorders of throat coordination find it difficult to protect the airway when they swallow, which can result in the aspiration of secretions.

(34) (A) Misses his medication.

Hyperglycemia is seen in diabetic patients. However, the blood sugar can be well controlled if the patient adheres to medications and lifestyle modifications. Patients with diabetes may develop moderate to severe hyperglycemia if they miss their medications.

(35) (D) To treat urinary tract infections.

An indwelling catheter is not used to treat urinary tract infections (UTIs). Instead, indwelling catheters are used for various other reasons, such as during surgery, for postoperative use, and to relieve urinary obstruction. In surgery and postoperative care, catheters are used to manage urinary output when patients are unable to use the bathroom themselves. They are also used to relieve urinary obstruction, and provide a way for urine to exit the bladder when normal urination is not possible.

(36) (B) Validate the woman's concerns and express empathy.

Patients with difficulties coping with losses and adjustment are encouraged to honestly express their feelings, needs, fears, and anxieties. It's important for medical personnel to validate such patients' concerns and be empathetic.

(37) (C) Physiological needs.

In Maslow's Hierarchy of Needs, the most relevant level for a 25-year-old client who is homeless and lacks access to food, water, or shelter is the physiological needs. Maslow's hierarchy is a psychological theory that prioritizes human needs in a pyramid, with the most basic needs at the bottom. The foundation of the pyramid is physiological needs, which include essential requirements for survival such as food, water, warmth, and rest.

(38) (A) Alzheimer's disease.

Alzheimer's disease is the most common type of dementia, accounting for about 60 to 70% of cases. It is a progressive neurodegenerative disease that causes the destruction of brain cells and the loss of cognitive function. The most common early symptoms of Alzheimer's disease are memory loss and difficulty with language. Other symptoms can include difficulty with problem-solving, judgment, and orientation.

(39) (D) Stay silent, as people may not understand their speech patterns.

This is incorrect. Elderly patients should be encouraged to speak up and express themselves without fear of being misunderstood.

(40) (C) Provide support and gently encourage communication about their condition.

When a patient is in denial about their medical condition, you should approach the situation with empathy and understanding. It's important to provide support and gently encourage the patient to express their feelings and concerns about their condition.

(41) (D) All of the above.

CNAs who work in the radiological unit should undergo regular checks for exposure levels. They should only be exposed to radiation when absolutely necessary and must always wear PPE in the unit.

(42) (D) All of the above.

As people age, the skin begins to dry out, and there is a constriction of blood vessels that affect the blood supply to the skin and limbs. Therefore, the skin is vulnerable to tears. Heart failure and falls are also major risk factors.

(43) (D) All of the above.

All of these are critical to the prevention of falls. CNAs should stay with such patients until they are done in the restroom. These patients should also be consistently observed, as they can easily fall.

(44) (D) Allergies.

Allergies can happen to any age group, but they are usually not associated with falls. Allergies occur when a person comes in contact with a substance that triggers an immune, inflammatory event, which can be mild or severe.

(45) (D) All of the above.

A CNA should know the history of patients, immediately categorize them as high risk for falls, and work with other health professionals in the management of patients.

(46) (A) Distraction.

Distraction redirects the mind from the current activity or emotions. In this case, the TV show helped redirect the patient's restlessness.

(47) (A) They allow control of access.

Entry supervision systems are placed in common areas of the nursing home to control who has access to enter. This ensures that only approved medical personnel or staff can access certain areas. This prevents ethical issues.

(48) (B) Handrails.

Handrails are one of the easiest places to pick up germs and infections because many people use them, but they can be overlooked when a facility is cleaned.

(49) (C) Joints are held together by tendons.

Joints are held together by ligaments. Tendons attach muscles to the bone at either the origin point or insertion point of the muscle.

(50) (C) Vitamin D deficiency.

In osteomalacia, there is a prolonged deficiency of vitamin D, which results in a softening of the bones. Calcium deficiency is seen in rickets and osteoporosis.

(51) (A) White blood cells.

White blood cells are responsible for the body's defenses. White blood cells can either be T-cells or B-cells. T-cells are responsible for cell-mediated immunity, while B-cells are responsible for humoral immunity.

(52) (A) Oxygenated blood.

The pulmonary vein carries oxygenated blood, which is a unique characteristic in the circulatory system. Veins carry deoxygenated blood from the body back to the heart. However, the pulmonary vein is an exception to this rule. It carries oxygen-rich blood from the lungs to the left atrium of the heart. This oxygenated blood is then distributed throughout the body via systemic circulation.

(53) (B) Fluids.

A patient suffering from diarrhea needs more fluids. Diarrhea can cause significant fluid loss, which increases the risk of dehydration. It's essential to replace these lost fluids to maintain hydration and proper body function. Although nutrients like proteins and vitamins are important for overall health and recovery, the immediate concern with diarrhea is the loss of fluids and electrolytes.

(54) (B) The pia mater.

The pia mater is directly situated on the brain.

(55) (A) TIA.

The symptoms described are most likely due to a transient ischemic attack, which mimics the presentations of a stroke but occurs briefly, with symptoms that are usually resolved spontaneously. TIAs should be managed promptly to prevent the occurrence of a stroke.

(56) (D) Rub the fingernails against the palm of the opposite hand.

The fingernails of one hand are cleaned by rubbing them against the palm of the opposite hand.

(57) (A) Handwashing.

If a patient continually reports diarrhea associated with diet, most likely it is a hygiene problem, and one of the first places to start management is to teach the patient how to wash his hands properly.

(58) (C) Start from the fingertips.

During handwashing, hands should be dried starting from the fingertips. The rationale behind this technique is to prevent contamination of the cleaned areas. The fingertips and areas between the fingers are more prone to microbial contamination due to their frequent use and contact with various surfaces. By drying from the fingertips and moving towards the wrists, there's a reduced risk of recontaminating the fingers.

(59) (C) Varicose veins.

Varicose veins refer to engorged, dilated, or enlarged veins that are usually formed as a result of the backflow of blood in the vein. They often occur in people who stand for hours at a time.

(60) (D) All of the above.

When applying a stocking, the foot of the stocking should be placed over the toes, foot, and heel. The process involves sliding the stocking over the toes first, then ensuring it covers the entire foot, and finally making sure it fits well over the heel.

(61) (B) At the waist.

When moving a patient, a CNA should place the transfer belt at the patient's waist. The transfer belt is also known as a gait belt, and it is used to help safely assist a patient who needs help with moving or walking.

(62) (B) After movement.

The transfer belt should be removed after the movement has been completed and the patient has returned to bed.

(63) (B) Not pull the patient with the transfer belt.

When moving a patient from the bed to a chair, a CNA should not pull the patient using the transfer belt. The transfer belt is designed to provide support and stability, not to be used as a tool to pull or drag a patient. Pulling a patient with the transfer belt can cause injury, discomfort, and can be unsafe.

(64) (B) Assisting with mobility and comfort due to increased body size.

At 40 weeks, a pregnancy is considered full-term, and the patient may experience significant discomfort due to increased body size and other late-stage pregnancy symptoms. A nurse aide's role would include assisting with mobility, providing comfort measures, and ensuring the patient's safety. This can involve helping with position changes, walking, and performing daily activities safely.

(65) (C) Not to contaminate the bedpan.

When assisting a patient with a bedpan, CNA Lee should pay special attention to not contaminating the bedpan. Ensuring that the bedpan remains clean and free from contamination is important for maintaining hygiene and preventing the spread of infection.

(66) (D) Bedsheets.

Privacy should be provided through the use of a curtain, door, or screen while the client uses a bedpan. Bedsheets are not appropriate for this purpose.

(67) (A) When the patient is experiencing difficulty breathing.

Raising the head of the bed can be very beneficial for patients who are having trouble breathing, as it allows for easier expansion of the chest and better oxygenation. This position is referred to as the Fowler's position, and it is commonly used for patients with respiratory issues, including those with pneumonia, chronic obstructive pulmonary disease (COPD), or congestive heart failure.

(68) (A) To monitor a patient's hydration and kidney function.

Accurate urine measurement is an important task for nurse aides as it provides vital information about a patient's hydration status and kidney function. Measuring urine output helps in detecting conditions like dehydration, kidney failure, or urinary tract issues.

(69) (D) All of the above.

Any condition that leads to the loss or destruction of teeth might be an indication for the use of dentures. Gum disease, intraoral cancer, and oral trauma might require dentures.

(70) (D) A and B.

Dentures should be rinsed in moderate-temperature running water before they are brushed. They should also be rinsed after they are brushed with toothpaste.

Test 3: Questions

(1) A 64-year-old patient with type 2 diabetes mellitus and hypertension is admitted to the medical ward. The patient is being managed for diabetic ketoacidosis. The CNA notices that the patient's saturation has dropped below the normal range. What should the CNA do?

(A) Perform CPR.

(B) Give intranasal oxygen.

(C) Escalate to the staff nurse.

(D) Escalate to the managing physician.

(2) What is a right of a patient in a healthcare facility?

(A) Right to abuse healthcare workers.

(B) Right to give orders to healthcare workers.

(C) Right to receive any treatment.

(D) Right to be treated with dignity.

(3) Eleven-year-old Mary suffers a burn injury to her face and is admitted to the burn unit. Her school friends are scheduled to visit her soon, and Mary worries she is now ugly. Which of the following needs should be provided for her?

(A) Social.

(B) Spiritual.

(C) Psychological.

(D) Physical.

(4) How do you write five in the afternoon on a 24-hour clock?

(A) 17:00.

(B) 5:00 p.m.

(C) 1500 p.m.

(D) 1700 p.m.

(5) What is an example of good body mechanics?

(A) Balance.

(B) Gait.

(C) Movement.

(D) Motion.

(6) A 68-year-old man suffers an acute ischemic stroke and is admitted to the neurology ward for treatment. What is a clinical sign of stroke?

(A) Fever.

(B) Dyspnea.

(C) Orthopnea.

(D) Muscle weakness.

(7) A 60-year-old patient with Alzheimer's dementia is admitted to the ward for treatment. She needs to eat in bed. Which device will make this easier for her?

(A) Bed cradle.

(B) Blanket.

(C) Over-bed table.

(D) Footpad.

(8) A 35-year-old is admitted to the medical ward for treatment of an acute kidney injury. The staff nurse delegates the CNA to measure the patient's urine output hourly. What will make this measurement easier?

(A) Urinary catheter.

(B) Hydrometer.

(C) Measuring table.

(D) Hourly urination.

(9) Which of the following is true about pain?

(A) It is a subjective experience.

(B) It is an objective experience.

(C) Its exact level can be measured.

(D) It is not real.

(10) How can HIV be contracted?

(A) Body contact.

(B) Blood.

(C) Saliva.

(D) Handshakes.

(11) Dementia patients do not commonly:
(A) Sundown.
(B) Have apraxia.
(C) Hoard.
(D) Pace.

(12) What is an appropriate snack for a four-year-old child?
(A) Grapes.
(B) Carrot sticks.
(C) Applesauce.
(D) Hot dogs.

(13) A 10-year-old boy is brought to the clinic with complaints of inability to see from the back of the class. His vision improves after he is moved to the front of the class. What is the most likely diagnosis?
(A) Glaucoma.
(B) Astigmatism.
(C) Cataracts.
(D) Myopia.

(14) What kinds of fluids are used for rehydration?
(A) Hypotonic saline.
(B) Hypertonic saline.
(C) Dextrose water.
(D) Normal saline.

(15) The outermost layer of the skin is called the:
(A) Epidermis.
(B) Dermis.
(C) Hypodermis.
(D) Endodermis.

(16) Which of the following is a critical role of a nurse aide while caring for a patient with diabetes?
(A) Administer insulin injections.
(B) Modify the patient's prescribed diabetes medication.
(C) Monitor and record blood sugar levels as directed.
(D) Advise the patient on dietary changes.

(17) A patient with diabetic mellitus especially needs regular:
(A) Foot care.
(B) Face care.
(C) Hand care.
(D) Perineal care.

(18) A 65-year-old patient is diagnosed with malabsorption disorder. What is a symptom of the condition?
(A) Hard stools.
(B) Bloody stool.
(C) Mucoid stool.
(D) Bulky, malodorous stool that floats.

(19) Mrs. Roberts is a 56-year-old woman who has difficulty with communication due to a stroke. She is usually friendly, but when you try to help her out of her chair today, she frowns and tries to hit you. What should you do?
(A) Ignore the behavior because she may be frustrated.
(B) Identify that Mrs. Roberts may be in pain and report it to the nurse.
(C) Ask her what you need to do for her.
(D) Identify that she may need medication for her behavior.

(20) What words are not used to describe pain?
(A) Throbbing.
(B) Burning.
(C) Dull.
(D) Round.

(21) What is the purpose of a flow sheet in a healthcare setting?
(A) To provide entertainment to patients.
(B) To keep track of staff vacation days.
(C) To document a patient's daily care and condition.
(D) To record the hospital's financial transactions.

(22) What does diastolic pressure measure in a blood pressure reading?
(A) The pressure in the arteries when the heart is at rest between beats.
(B) The pressure in the arteries during exercise.
(C) The oxygen level in the blood.
(D) The number of heartbeats per minute.

(23) A 67-year-old woman is brought to the clinic for evaluation of recurrent tiredness. She is found to be malnourished. What is not a common reason for malnutrition?
(A) Financial issues.
(B) Fever.
(C) Inadequate absorption.
(D) Inadequate food consumption.

(24) Which patients most commonly have bladder outlet obstruction?
(A) Young males.
(B) Elderly females.
(C) Elderly males.
(D) Young females.

(25) Which measure is most beneficial to patients with urinary incontinence?
(A) Incontinence pads.
(B) Intravenous fluids.
(C) Antibiotics.
(D) Analgesics.

(26) What is not a nonverbal expression of pain?
(A) Frowns.
(B) Crying.
(C) Singing.
(D) Restlessness.

(27) A 56-year-old patient with limited arm movement attempts to eat. Which of the following utensils can help this patient?
(A) Normal utensils.
(B) Short utensils.
(C) Extension utensils.
(D) Plastic utensils.

(28) All of the following can influence a patient's choice of food except:
(A) Culture.
(B) Religion.
(C) Height.
(D) Ability to prepare food.

(29) What is not a manifestation of dementia?
(A) Amnesia.
(B) Aphasia.
(C) Apraxia.
(D) Delirium.

(30) What is the best practice when washing a patient's genital area?
(A) Use hot water to ensure all bacteria are killed.
(B) Wash from the least contaminated area to the most contaminated area.
(C) Wash only once a week to avoid skin irritation.
(D) Use the same cloth for the entire body for efficiency.

(31) Which of the following terminologies is incorrectly matched?
(A) Flexion – bend.
(B) Extension – straighten.
(C) Adduction – movement toward the body.
(D) Abduction – movement toward the body.

(32) A 58-year-old man with Parkinson's disease is admitted to the neurology ward. Which of the following problems should the CNA anticipate that the patient may have?
(A) Visual problems.
(B) Movement problems.
(C) Breathing problems.
(D) Fever.

(33) A 43-year-old man on admission for pneumonia develops respiratory distress. Which vital sign may indicate this problem?
(A) Temperature.
(B) Pulse.
(C) Respiratory rate.
(D) Blood pressure.

(34) A 56-year-old patient with dementia is found to have chronic kidney disease. In the later stages of the disease, what treatment might the patient need?
(A) Analgesics.
(B) Intravenous fluids.
(C) Chemotherapy.
(D) Dialysis.

(35) All of the following are used in the provision of nail care, except:
(A) Nail clippers.
(B) Emery board.
(C) Orange stick.
(D) Hand sanitizer.

(36) How should CNAs help patients who have a hard time coping with losses and adjustments?
(A) Listen to the patients' concerns but do not assure them adequate care will be provided.
(B) Listen to the patients and assure them that adequate care will be provided.
(C) First, assure the patients that adequate care will be provided. Then listen to them.
(D) Ignore the patients' concerns.

(37) What precautions should a nurse aide take when caring for a patient with measles?
(A) Use standard precautions only, as measles is not highly contagious.
(B) Implement droplet precautions and wear appropriate PPE.
(C) Isolate the patient in a room with high temperatures.
(D) Encourage frequent and close physical contact to build immunity.

(38) An 80-year-old woman is being cared for by a CNA. Which of the following symptoms do not need to be reported to the charge nurse or physician?
(A) Changes in mental status.
(B) Changes in awareness level.
(C) Decline in personal hygiene.
(D) Increased concern for hygiene.

(39) What is the recommended precaution when caring for a patient with chickenpox?
(A) Wear a standard surgical mask.
(B) Implement airborne precautions and use PPE.
(C) Increase room temperature significantly.
(D) Encourage the patient to exercise frequently.

(40) Alice is a CNA who recently came down with a respiratory tract infection when she worked in the respiratory unit. What kind of hazard was she exposed to?
(A) Radiation.
(B) Infectious diseases.
(C) Disinfection.
(D) Allergies.

(41) One way to cope with stress as a CNA is to:
(A) Delegate tasks when necessary.
(B) Try to finish all tasks alone.
(C) Work extra hours.
(D) Avoid work as much as possible.

(42) Which of the following patients is most prone to burns if a fire occurs in a healthcare facility?
(A) A patient in a wheelchair.
(B) An unconscious patient.
(C) A conscious patient.
(D) All of the above.

(43) Which patient is least likely to experience falls and injuries?
(A) A patient with diabetes.
(B) A patient with Alzheimer's.
(C) A patient with a respiratory tract infection.
(D) All of the above.

(44) A 55-year-old female patient is brought into the ER with complaints of unclear speech and weakness on her left side. What is the most probable diagnosis?
(A) Tuberculosis.
(B) Stroke.
(C) Epilepsy.
(D) Concussion.

(45) Which of the following are not relevant observations in fall assessment?
(A) Weakness.
(B) Edema.
(C) Anxiety.
(D) Sexual orientation.

(46) When should bedrails be set up for a patient at high risk of falls?
(A) Always.
(B) At noon.
(C) In the morning.
(D) At night.

(47) Which safety device beeps when patients wander out of the hospital premises?
(A) Emergency alert.
(B) Bed alarm.
(C) Wander guard.
(D) Bed rail.

(48) What is the role of a CNA who observes a patient's relatives throw litter on the floor during a visit?
(A) Send them out.
(B) Yell at them.
(C) Report their behavior to the senior nurse.
(D) Calmly educate them on hygienic practices during hospital visits.

(49) A 56-year-old woman complains of recurrent lower back pain and says that she feels shorter than she used to be. What is the most likely diagnosis?

(A) Osteomalacia.

(B) Fracture.

(C) Osteoporosis.

(D) All of the above.

(50) What is not one of the components of the blood?

(A) Erythrocytes.

(B) Leukocytes.

(C) Synovial fluid.

(D) Thrombocytes.

(51) A patient with low hematocrit is deficient in which blood cells?

(A) Red blood cells.

(B) White blood cells.

(C) Platelets.

(D) Lymphocytes.

(52) CNAs who manage patients who have breathlessness must:

(A) Ensure oxygen is available.

(B) Check the flow rate regularly.

(C) Ensure patients are in the proper position.

(D) All of the above.

(53) A patient with liver disease might present with generalized body swelling. What does this raise the risk of?

(A) Bed sores.

(B) Flu.

(C) Diarrhea.

(D) All of the above.

(54) How many major lobes are present in the brain?

(A) 2.

(B) 4.

(C) 6.

(D) 8.

(55) A CNA can help a patient who is in the recovery process from a stroke with:
(A) Mobility.
(B) Feeding.
(C) Hygiene.
(D) All of the above.

(56) What important step must CNA George take before any procedure is performed on a client?
(A) Explain the procedure.
(B) Introduce himself.
(C) Maintain eye contact.
(D) All of the above.

(57) What is an appropriate action for a nurse aide to take when caring for a patient experiencing constipation?
(A) Provide a high-fiber diet and encourage hydration.
(B) Advise the patient to ignore it as it will resolve on its own.
(C) Immediately give the patient a strong laxative without consulting a nurse.
(D) Restrict the patient's fluid intake to decrease bowel movements.

(58) What is a key action for a nurse aide when caring for a patient with diarrhea?
(A) Limit the patient's fluid intake to reduce stool volume.
(B) Encourage the patient to eat spicy food to settle the stomach.
(C) Provide clear liquids and encourage hydration to prevent dehydration.
(D) Advise the patient to hold in the diarrhea to strengthen bowel muscles.

(59) How long should a CNA count respiration for?
(A) 15 seconds.
(B) 30 seconds.
(C) 60 seconds.
(D) All of the above.

(60) What is one full respiration cycle?
(A) One inspiration.
(B) One inspiration, one expiration.
(C) Two inspirations.
(D) Two expirations.

(61) Before CNAs record specific data after physical interaction with a patient, they should:
(A) Ask the patient to briefly hold their breath.
(B) Count respirations again.
(C) Wash their hands.
(D) All of the above.

(62) How does a CNA correctly put on a gown?
(A) From the front.
(B) From the back.
(C) From the side.
(D) From above.

(63) When should gloves be put on?
(A) Before a gown.
(B) After a gown.
(C) After a gown is removed.
(D) All of the above.

(64) What should a nurse aide do if they find a patient smoking in a non-smoking area of a healthcare facility?
(A) Join the patient in smoking to build rapport.
(B) Politely remind the patient of the non-smoking policy.
(C) Ignore the behavior as addressing it is not within the nurse aide's scope of practice.
(D) Punish the patient by restricting their privileges.

(65) What kind of shirt might a male patient be dressed in?
(A) A blue shirt.
(B) A black shirt.
(C) A gray shirt.
(D) A shirt of his choice.

(66) How does a CNA prevent overexposure when he assists a patient while the patient is dressing?
(A) Ensure the patient is seated upright in bed.
(B) Ensure the patient eats well.
(C) Use the patient's towel.
(D) Ensure the patient's chest is well covered.

(67) How does a CNA dress a patient with left-sided body weakness?
(A) From the right side.
(B) From the left side.
(C) From the bottom.
(D) From any side.

(68) What portion of the foot is not dried in foot care?
(A) Top.
(B) Bottom.
(C) Between the toes.
(D) None.

(69) Which of the following is not needed in foot care?
(A) Basin.
(B) Signaling device.
(C) Towels.
(D) Clips.

(70) A CNA performs foot care. When should she remove her gloves?
(A) After the foot is washed.
(B) After the foot is dried.
(C) After the basin is put away.
(D) After all used materials are disposed of.

Test 3: Answers and Explanations

(1) (C) Escalate to the staff nurse.

A certified CNA may be delegated to check a patient's vital signs at intervals. Any deviations from normal should be escalated to the staff nurse. It is out of the scope of the CNA's responsibility in this case to attempt any procedure or management plan for the patient.

(2) (D) Right to be treated with dignity.

Every patient has a right to be treated with dignity. CNAs must ensure they protect patient's privacy and confidentiality. They must be guided by the core principles of medical ethics at all times.

(3) (C) Psychological.

This young patient with burns to the face needs psychological counseling. Oftentimes, patients with burns to the face are worried about being "ugly." This may cause them even more distress than the physical injury itself.

(4) (A) 17:00.

The 24-hour clock records the time in 24 hours rather than dividing the day into two. There is no need to add a.m. or p.m. to the time. One hour above 12 noon is recorded as 13:00, and this is continued up until midnight.

(5) (A) Balance.

Because part of the job requirement of CNAs is to assist in the transfer of patients, they need to learn good body mechanics to prevent injury. Body mechanics include balance, coordination, etc.

(6) (D) Muscle weakness.

Stroke is a cerebrovascular disease that is characterized by sudden onset of neurological impairment due to cerebral, spinal, or retinal ischemia. The neurological damage manifests as muscle weakness and paralysis. In addition, there may be speech difficulties and sensory abnormalities.

(7) (C) Over-bed table.

The over-bed table is a device used to help patients who cannot move out of bed. The table is used to support food. The foot pad, blanket, and bed cradle are not used to support food.

(8) (A) Urinary catheter.

The urinary catheter is a device that is passed through the urethra to the bladder to facilitate drainage of urine to the exterior. One of the indications for a urinary catheter is a condition that requires adequate monitoring of urinary output, such as acute kidney injury.

(9) (A) It is a subjective experience.

Pain is a subjective experience characterized by a physical, emotional, or psychological response to a noxious stimulus. There is no objective way to measure pain. However, there are scales to extrapolate the degree of pain. Pain is a real experience and should be taken seriously.

(10) (B) Blood.

HIV is a viral disease that is transmitted by sexual intercourse, contact with infected blood and blood products, and body fluids. The disease is common in drug abusers, homosexuals, and other high-risk populations.

(11) (B) Have apraxia.

Apraxia is the inability to perform the steps necessary to complete a task despite a person having the ability and desire to perform the task.

(12) (C) Applesauce.

The American Academy of Pediatricians recommends that young children not be given round, firm foods such as peanuts, hot dogs, and carrot sticks unless they are chopped into small pieces no larger than half an inch.

(13) (D) Myopia.

Myopia is a refractive eye condition also known as short-sightedness. It occurs as a result of increased length or convexity of the crystalline lens. The image formed is in front of the retina. Thus, objects close to the eyes are seen clearly, while objects far away appear blurry.

(14) (D) Normal saline.

Dehydration is a common presentation seen in patients. It may occur from gastroenteritis, vomiting, excessive sweating, etc. Treatment is the replacement of body fluids with normal saline or ringer's lactate.

(15) (A) Epidermis.

The epidermis is the outermost layer of the skin. It is divided into different strata, each with specific characteristics. The stratum corneum is the outermost layer of the epidermis. It protects the underlying tissue from damage. A breach of the epidermis exposes the skin to infection.

(16) (C) Monitor and record blood sugar levels as directed.

For a patient with diabetes, a key responsibility is to monitor and record the patient's blood sugar levels. This is essential for managing the patient's condition and ensuring that any necessary adjustments to their care plan can be made promptly.

(17) (A) Foot care.

Patients with diabetes mellitus are at increased risk of diabetic foot ulcers, which are sometimes limb-threatening or life-threatening. Prevention of foot ulcers is one of the main goals of management. One of the ways to achieve this is regular foot care.

(18) (D) Bulky, malodorous stool that floats.

Malabsorption syndromes are a group of disorders characterized by an inability to digest and absorb nutrients from food. A common presentation of most disorders is loose stool that floats.

(19) (B) Identify that Mrs. Roberts may be in pain and report it to the nurse.

Refusal of care and frowns are nonverbal expressions of pain. A CNA should recognize these signs and report them to the nurse.

(20) (D) Round.

Common terminologies used to describe pain include throbbing, burning, dull, aching, sharp, piercing, stabbing, tingling, pins-and-needles sensation, squeezing, crushing or feeling of pressure, pulsating or pounding, nagging, gnawing, cramping, or spasms. "Round" is not a common term used to describe pain.

(21) (C) To document a patient's daily care and condition.

A flow sheet is an important tool used for the systematic and concise recording of a patient's care and condition over a period of time. It includes vital signs, fluid intake and output, medications administered, and other relevant care details.

(22) (A) The pressure in the arteries when the heart is at rest between beats.

Diastolic pressure is the lower number in a blood pressure reading and reflects the pressure in the arteries when the heart is resting between beats. It is a critical indicator of cardiovascular health, and a high diastolic pressure could potentially indicate an increased risk for heart-related issues.

(23) (B) Fever.

Although fever can cause weight loss if it continues for a long time, most people with short febrile episodes don't develop malnutrition. However, financial issues, problems with gastrointestinal absorption of digested food, and inadequate eating can all contribute to malnutrition. Other causes of malnutrition are chronic diseases.

(24) (C) Elderly males.

Bladder outlet obstruction is more common in elderly males due to benign prostatic hyperplasia. The risk of benign prostatic hyperplasia increases with age. More than half of men have an enlarged prostate by age 70.

(25) (A) Incontinence pads.

Incontinence pads help to prevent patients from soiling themselves and their clothing. Incontinence pads should be changed regularly to reduce the risk of ammoniacal dermatitis and UTIs

(26) (C) Singing.

Frowning, groaning, crying, and restlessness are all nonverbal ways patients use to communicate pain.

(27) (C) Extension utensils.

Extension utensils are used by patients who struggle to reach their mouths with normal-sized utensils. Extension utensils are adjustable and can be adapted to fit different patient requirements.

(28) (C) Height.

Height does not influence a patient's choice of food.

(29) (D) Delirium.

Delirium is not a feature of dementia. Dementia is a chronic progressive disorder characterized by degeneration in a patient's memory and intellect. It can be associated with amnesia (memory loss). Other presentations include apraxia, agnosia, and aphasia.

(30) (B) Wash from the least contaminated area to the most contaminated area.

When washing a patient's genital area, it is important to start from the least contaminated area and move towards the most contaminated area. This practice helps prevent the spread of bacteria and reduces the risk of urinary tract infections, especially in females. The water used should be warm, not hot, to avoid burning or irritating the skin.

(31) (D) Abduction – movement toward the body.

Flexion describes the bending of body parts across a joint. Extension is the straightening of body parts across a joint. Abduction is the movement of a body part away from the body, while adduction is the movement toward the body.

(32) (B) Movement problems.

A patient with Parkinson's disease most likely has tremors and postural instability like festinant or shuffling gait. Parkinson's disease is a neurological disorder that is characterized by tremors, bradykinesia, and rigidity. Some patients also have autonomic symptoms.

(33) (C) Respiratory rate.

The respiratory rate is a vital sign that may indicate the cause of new-onset respiratory distress in a patient.

(34) (D) Dialysis.

Dialysis is a form of renal replacement therapy used in patients with end-stage renal failure. It is used to remove toxic materials and waste products of metabolism from the blood.

(35) (D) Hand sanitizer.

When providing nail care, a hand sanitizer is not generally used as a tool. Nail care generally involves tools like nail clippers for trimming nails, an emery board for smoothing and shaping the nails, and an orange stick for cleaning under the nails and pushing back cuticles.

(36) (B) Listen to the patients and assure them that adequate care will be provided.

When assisting patients who are struggling with coping with losses and adjustments, CNAs should listen to the patients' concerns and assure them that adequate care will be provided. Listening empathetically to patients' concerns is a critical aspect of providing emotional support and building trust. It allows patients to express their feelings and feel heard, which is important in coping with difficult situations.

(37) (B) Implement droplet precautions and wear appropriate PPE.

Measles is a highly contagious viral infection that spreads through respiratory droplets when an infected person coughs or sneezes. When caring for a patient with measles, nurse aides should implement droplet precautions, which include wearing masks, gowns, and gloves, and possibly using a face shield or goggles if there is a risk of droplet exposure to the eyes.

(38) (D) Increased concern for hygiene.

CNAs should take note of changes in mental status, awareness levels, and decline in personal hygiene. These changes must be reported to the physician in charge, who can diagnose medical conditions and direct the appropriate line of care.

(39) (B) Implement airborne precautions and use PPE.

Chickenpox is caused by the varicella-zoster virus, and it is highly contagious. It can be spread through both direct contact and airborne transmission. When caring for a patient with chickenpox, nurse aides should implement airborne precautions, which include wearing appropriate PPE such as N95 masks, gowns, and gloves. They should also ensure that the patient is in an appropriate isolated room if available.

(40) (B) Infectious diseases.

Alice is a CNA working in a respiratory unit, and likely contracted a respiratory tract infection due to exposure to infectious diseases, which is common in healthcare settings, particularly in units dealing with respiratory conditions. Respiratory units often treat patients with infections that can be transmitted through the air or close contact.

(41) (A) Delegate tasks when necessary.

Delegation is a way to reduce stress or burdens. However, tasks must be delegated based on competence and skill.

(42) (B) An unconscious patient.

Unconscious patients are most prone to burns in the event of a fire outbreak because they cannot move out of harm's way.

(43) (C) A patient with a respiratory tract infection.

A patient with a respiratory tract infection is unlikely to experience a fall or injury. Patients with diabetes may have poor sensation in the feet due to nerve damage, and if they walk around barefoot, they might not be able to feel sharp objects or notice when they are injured. Patients with Alzheimer's may have problems with navigation. All these increase the possibility of a fall in these patients.

(44) (B) Stroke.

Stroke presents with slurred or unclear speech and body weakness that is localized to one side. CNAs must be able to recognize these symptoms so they can either advise the patient or act swiftly to inform the appropriate healthcare personnel.

(45) (D) Sexual orientation.

In a fall assessment, sexual orientation is not a relevant factor to consider. Fall assessments focus on physical, psychological, and environmental factors that could increase the risk of falls. These include issues like muscle weakness, which can affect mobility and balance; edema, or swelling, which can indicate underlying health issues that might impact stability; and anxiety, which can affect a person's ability to move safely and confidently.

(46) (A) Always.

Bedrails are a safety measure used to prevent patients from accidentally rolling or falling out of bed. In the case of patients who are at a high risk of falling, such as those with mobility issues, confusion, or certain medical conditions, it is important to have bedrails up continuously. This ensures their safety throughout the day and night, regardless of the time.

(47) (C) Wander guard.

Wander guards are electronic devices that beep when patients wander into areas that are hazardous within or outside the hospital premises. Staff members are alerted and can provide prompt intervention to ensure the safety of patients.

(48) (D) Calmly educate them on hygienic practices during hospital visits.

If a patient's relatives litter, they should be educated about the need for a clean environment for the patients and shown where the trash cans are.

(49) (C) Osteoporosis.

Osteoporosis is a disease that occurs due to an imbalance between bone formation and bone destruction, such that more bone cells are destroyed than formed. The result is weakened bones, which leads to fractures, lower back pain, reduction in height, bone deformities, and gums that recede.

(50) (C) Synovial fluid.

The synovial fluid is a component of the joint capsule, not of the blood. It serves as a lubricant to prevent friction of articular ends of bones during movement.

(51) (A) Red blood cells.

The value of the hematocrit is a measure of the red blood cells in the body. A patient that has a low hematocrit has a low red blood cell count.

(52) (D) All of the above.

In patients suffering from breathlessness, correct positioning aids breathing and clears fluids in the lungs. Oxygen must be available, and the flow rate should be regularly checked.

(53) (A) Bed sores.

A patient with liver disease complicated by swelling will need help to move around. Due to their inability to move around, the patient might develop bedsores if left for too long without turning.

(54) (B) 4.

There are four brain lobes—the frontal, the posterior, the temporal, and the parietal.

(55) (D) All of the above.

A patient who had a stroke might need help with feeding, movement, and hygiene. The extent of assistance needed will depend on the level of illness.

(56) (D) All of the above.

Before the start of any procedure, CNAs must introduce themselves and explain details about the procedure to the client in clear, simple, and direct terms. Eye contact should be maintained while the explanation is given.

(57) (A) Provide a high-fiber diet and encourage hydration.

For a patient experiencing constipation, a nurse aide should assist in providing a diet high in fiber (if allowed by the patient's care plan) and encourage the patient to drink plenty of fluids. Fiber helps to bulk up stools and promote regular bowel movements, while adequate hydration helps keep the stools soft. This approach is often effective in managing constipation.

(58) (C) Provide clear liquids and encourage hydration to prevent dehydration.

Diarrhea can cause rapid fluid loss and put patients at risk of dehydration. It is important for a nursing assistant to encourage the patient to consume clear liquids, like water, broth, and electrolyte solutions, to maintain hydration. This helps to replace fluids that are lost due to diarrhea and supports overall patient health.

(59) (C) 60 seconds.

The standard respiration count is 60 seconds.

(60) (B) One inspiration, one expiration.

One full respiration cycle consists of one inspiration (inhaling) followed by one expiration (exhaling). This cycle represents the complete process of taking air into the lungs (inspiration) and then expelling it (expiration). It is the basic unit of measurement for respiratory rate and function.

(61) (C) Wash their hands.

CNAs should always wash their hands before recording the results of any examination or making contact with a patient. The rationale behind this is that if records are written or typed, the CNA does not transfer germs or bacteria to either the pen or keyboard.

(62) (B) From the back.

When a CNA puts on a gown as part of personal protective equipment, the correct way is to do so from the back. The gown should be approached and picked up by the edges near the neck ties without touching the outside surface. The CNA then slips their arms into the sleeves, and the gown is secured at the neck and waist, which ensures full coverage of their clothing.

(63) (B) After a gown.

Gloves should be put on after donning a gown when following proper personal protective equipment protocol. The sequence is important to maintain the sterility and effectiveness of the PPE. First, the gown is put on to cover clothing and protect skin from contamination. After the gown is securely in place, gloves are worn. The gloves should overlap the gown's cuffs to ensure a continuous barrier of protection. This sequence reduces the risk of contaminating the gloves when putting on the gown.

(64) (B) Politely remind the patient of the non-smoking policy.

It is important for a nurse aide to maintain a safe and healthy environment for all patients and staff in the healthcare facility. If a patient is found smoking in a non-smoking area, the nurse aide should politely remind them of the facility's smoking policies and assist them in locating a designated smoking area if there is one available.

(65) (D) A shirt of his choice.

When dressing a male patient, the most appropriate option is to allow him to wear a shirt of his choice, assuming he is able to make that decision. This choice respects the patient's autonomy and personal preferences and contributes to his sense of dignity and individuality.

(66) (D) Ensure the patient's chest is well-covered.

When CNAs help patients to dress, they should always ensure that the chest and other sensitive parts are well covered.

(67) (A) From the right side.

When dressing a patient with left-sided body weakness, a CNA should start by dressing the weaker (left) side first. This means that they should put the patient's left arm or leg through the clothing before the right arm or leg. Dressing the weaker side first helps to minimize the amount of movement and effort required from the patient and can be less painful for them.

(68) (D) None.

All parts of the feet should be dried. This includes the top, bottom, and especially between the toes. The area between the toes should always be kept dry to prevent the growth of fungus, bacteria, or yeast.

(69) (D) Clips.

A basin is needed to hold water to wash the feet. Towels are needed to clean the feet and dry them. A signaling device should always be within reach of the patient in case assistance is needed. Clips are unnecessary.

(70) (D) After all used materials are disposed of.

Throughout the whole process, the CNA should wear gloves. The gloves should only be disposed of after the procedure is complete.

Test 4: Questions

(1) During ward rounds, an LPN tells the CNA to regularly turn a 75-year-old diabetic man admitted to the ward for foot ulcer treatment. This LPN used the principle of:
(A) Delegation.
(B) Mediation.
(C) Orders.
(D) Assignment.

(2) What should a nursing assistant do when assisting with bladder training for a patient?
(A) Increase the patient's fluid intake dramatically to encourage frequent urination.
(B) Set a regular schedule for toileting to establish bladder control.
(C) Advise the patient to avoid using the bathroom until absolutely necessary.
(D) Recommend herbal supplements to improve bladder function.

(3) A CNA does not respond quickly to a patient who calls for help. Which of the following needs of the patient were not met?
(A) Sexual.
(B) Physical.
(C) Safety.
(D) Self-esteem.

(4) Which principle of medical ethics protects the patient against harm from a healthcare provider's intervention?
(A) Justice.
(B) Integrity.
(C) Nonmaleficence.
(D) Autonomy.

(5) A 25-year-old with a history of drug use disorder is brought to the ER. He is confused and combative, and the managing team considers the use of restraints. Which of the following is true about restraints?
(A) They must never be used.
(B) Physical restraints should be released regularly.
(C) Only chemical restraints can be used.
(D) Only physical restraints can be used.

(6) A 44-year-old overweight patient wants to be screened for diabetes because of her family history. Which of the following values of fasting blood sugar is used to diagnose diabetes?

(A) Greater than 6.0.

(B) Greater than 7.0.

(C) Greater than 8.0.

(D) Greater than 5.0.

(7) A 16-year-old had an appendectomy and is to be moved to the recovery room on a stretcher. What is the best bed for this patient?

(A) Surgical bed.

(B) Open bed.

(C) Closed bed.

(D) Empty bed.

(8) The term nil per os (NPO) means:

(A) No food or fluids.

(B) No fluids.

(C) No food but can take fluids.

(D) Nothing by mouth.

(9) Which of the following is true about chronic pain?

(A) It lasts longer than six months.

(B) It lasts less than six months.

(C) It lasts less than a month.

(D) It includes any pain felt for more than a week.

(10) Which investigation can be used to diagnose stroke?

(A) Computed tomography.

(B) X-ray.

(C) Bone scan.

(D) Fasting blood sugar.

(11) Mrs. Elizabeth has been diagnosed with dementia. She asks the same questions repeatedly. Which of the following is not appropriate behavior for a medical practitioner who attends to this patient?
(A) Remind the patient her questions have already been answered.
(B) Be empathetic with the patient.
(C) Be patient with the patient.
(D) Answer all the patient's questions.

(12) A CNA must care for patients of all ages. Which of the following age groups is likely to be afraid of the dark?
(A) Infants.
(B) Toddlers.
(C) Preschoolers.
(D) School-age children.

(13) A 70-year-old woman develops sensorineural hearing loss, which gets progressively worse with age. What is the most likely cause of her hearing loss?
(A) Presbycusis.
(B) Wax impaction.
(C) Otitis media.
(D) Trauma.

(14) Which of the following is true about asthma?
(A) It is an acute condition.
(B) It is a chronic disease.
(C) The initial treatment is oxygen therapy.
(D) It occurs mainly in the elderly.

(15) A 70-year-old patient developed low back pain five years ago. He was subsequently diagnosed with lumbar spondylosis. His pain has worsened recently. This type of pain is referred to as:
(A) Acute pain.
(B) Chronic pain.
(C) Mild pain.
(D) Tenderness.

(16) A 33-year-old man is to be moved to the operating room in a wheelchair. In which of the following positions should the patient be to facilitate easy transfer to the wheelchair?

(A) Edge of the bed.

(B) Head of the bed.

(C) Foot of the bed.

(D) Center of the bed.

(17) What is an appropriate approach for a nursing assistant when caring for a patient with Alzheimer's disease?

(A) Engage in argumentative conversations to stimulate the patient's thinking.

(B) Use physical restraints to prevent the patient from wandering.

(C) Maintain a routine, calm, and familiar environment.

(D) Frequently change the patient's surroundings to provide variety.

(18) Which of the following classes of food helps build muscle and repair damaged cells?

(A) Carbohydrates.

(B) Oils.

(C) Proteins.

(D) Fats.

(19) A CNA is about to apply an ice bag to Mrs. Roland's left foot when he notices the foot is cold to touch and has purplish discoloration. What should the CNA do?

(A) Explain the procedure to Mrs. Roland, and then proceed to apply the ice.

(B) Apply warmth instead because her foot is already cold.

(C) Ask the patient where she wants the ice to be placed.

(D) Immediately report the observation to the nurse.

(20) It's 2:30 a.m., and Mr. James complains to the CNA that he can't sleep. How can the CNA help this patient?

(A) Apply heat to relieve any pain.

(B) Sit and talk with him for a while.

(C) Suggest that Mr. James take another dose of his medication.

(D) Apply ice to relieve any pain.

(21) Mr. Peters is a 96-year-old man. He tells the CNA he has lived a good life and he is ready to go home when his good Lord takes him. This is an expression of:
(A) Resignation.
(B) Hope.
(C) Acceptance.
(D) Denial.

(22) Excessive worry is referred to as:
(A) Generalized anxiety disorder.
(B) Phobia.
(C) Depression.
(D) Social phobia.

(23) A 72-year-old man with chronic inflammatory bowel disease and malnutrition is brought to the clinic to establish dietary care. Which diet prescription is most appropriate for the patient?
(A) Therapeutic diet.
(B) Early diet.
(C) Full diet.
(D) Dash diet.

(24) A 70-year-old patient develops urinary retention. He has a history of benign prostatic hyperplasia. A CNA should:
(A) Do a urethral catheterization.
(B) Administer analgesics.
(C) Encourage him to push the urine out.
(D) Use intravenous fluids to flush the urine out.

(25) Which of the following should be reported to the nurse if seen in a patient?
(A) Cloudy and smelly urine.
(B) 400 mls of urine passed at once.
(C) 500 mls of urine passed at once.
(D) Urination every five hours.

(26) A 30-year-old who recently underwent an appendectomy complains of pain one day after surgery. Which of the following actions by the CNA is most appropriate?

(A) Give acetaminophen.

(B) Give oral morphine.

(C) Give diazepam.

(D) Inform the nurse on duty.

(27) A 64-year-old patient constantly spills when he drinks from a cup. Which of the following can benefit the patient?

(A) Commercial straw holder.

(B) Plastic cup.

(C) Glass cup.

(D) Stainless steel cup.

(28) What should CNAs do first after they assist patients with elimination?

(A) Wash their hands.

(B) Transfer the patient.

(C) Counsel the patient.

(D) Document the procedure.

(29) Amnesia is a term used to describe:

(A) Memory loss.

(B) Memory gain.

(C) Energy loss.

(D) Speech loss.

(30) Which of the following is true about dementia and delirium?

(A) Delirium is insidious in onset.

(B) Dementia is sudden in onset.

(C) Dementia occurs most commonly in young people.

(D) Delirium can be triggered by infections.

(31) What is an important consideration when providing care to a patient with arthritis?
(A) Encourage the patient to remain immobile to reduce pain.
(B) Assist with gentle range-of-motion exercises as recommended.
(C) Apply cold compresses to the joints at all times.
(D) Discourage the use of any pain medication.

(32) Multiple sclerosis is best described as a:
(A) Neurological disease.
(B) Cardiovascular disease.
(C) Gastrointestinal diseases.
(D) Skeletal disease.

(33) A 56-year-old patient undergoes abdominal surgery for acute cholecystitis. She is in the postoperative ward and is doing well. Which measure can reduce the risk of atelectasis in this patient?
(A) Chest compression.
(B) Regular exercise.
(C) Regular meals.
(D) Incentive spirometry.

(34) What is not a presentation of chronic kidney disease?
(A) Anemia.
(B) Fatigue.
(C) Swollen face.
(D) Polycythemia.

(35) A CNA notices a patient's nails are thick and unusually convex. What is the next best action?
(A) Ignore the issue.
(B) Inform the nurse.
(C) Remove the whole nail.
(D) Collect a nail specimen for investigation.

(36) The roles of a CNA include all of the following except:
(A) Help patients adjust and build interactions with other individuals.
(B) Help patients participate in daily routines.
(C) Help patients financially as the need arises.
(D) Educate patients on the importance of care, hygiene, and good relationships.

(37) It is difficult for a 45-year-old client to meet his basic needs, such as food and shelter. How can a CNA help this client?
(A) Report the client's case to the police.
(B) Force the client to get a job.
(C) Help the client get basic needs from another client.
(D) Help the client connect with resources such as food banks, homeless shelters, and government assistance programs.

(38) How should you assist a patient experiencing back pain?
(A) Encourage complete bed rest for several days.
(B) Help the patient with prescribed exercises and proper body mechanics.
(C) Advise the patient to lift heavy objects to strengthen the back.
(D) Ignore the pain as it is a common issue that does not require attention.

(39) A 65-year-old woman presents to the clinic. She reports that she feels lonely and isolated lately. She says that she has lost touch with many of her friends and doesn't spend as much time with her family as she used to. What is the most likely reason for this patient's relationship changes?
(A) Normal changes in aging.
(B) Retirement.
(C) Death of a spouse.
(D) Move to a new city.

(40) In which area is sterilization most important?
(A) The emergency room.
(B) The nursing ward.
(C) The operating room.
(D) The kitchen.

(41) What is an appropriate action to take when caring for a patient experiencing a severe migraine?

(A) Expose the patient to bright lights to reduce the severity of the migraine.

(B) Provide a quiet and dark environment to help alleviate symptoms.

(C) Encourage the patient to perform high-intensity exercises.

(D) Insist the patient watch television to distract from the pain.

(42) A 50-year-old female patient had a partial stroke. How can a CNA help prevent bedsores in this patient?

(A) Feed the patient frequently.

(B) Clean the patient regularly.

(C) Turn the patient frequently.

(D) Immobilize the patient.

(43) A 70-year-old man with a right leg fracture needs help in many areas except when he:

(A) Eats.

(B) Speaks.

(C) Takes a bath.

(D) Uses the restroom.

(44) If a CNA is stressed, what are the possible complications?

(A) Lower output.

(B) Poor job performance.

(C) Absenteeism.

(D) All of the above.

(45) Why are restraints important in a healthcare setting?

(A) To silence a loud patient.

(B) To prevent break-ins.

(C) As a first-line method to ensure compliance.

(D) As a last resort to prevent harm to patients or others.

(46) When chemical restraints are used, this must be:
(A) Documented.
(B) Explained.
(C) Ignored.
(D) All of the above.

(47) Which of the following is not correct about restraints?
(A) They can be physical or chemical.
(B) They can be used to restrict patient movements.
(C) They're illegal.
(D) They're useful in the prevention of violent behavior.

(48) Which of these diseases does not carry the risk of airborne transmission in a healthcare facility?
(A) Tuberculosis.
(B) Chickenpox.
(C) Measles.
(D) Bartonella.

(49) What is a joint?
(A) A unit of movement.
(B) A collection of bones and muscles.
(C) Where two or more bones meet.
(D) All of the above.

(50) A patient presents with a low platelet count. What is the patient most at risk of?
(A) Blood clots.
(B) Pulmonary embolism.
(C) Bleeding.
(D) All of the above.

(51) If a patient suffers from anemia, what should a CNA watch out for?
(A) Falls.
(B) Fainting.
(C) Breathlessness.
(D) All of the above.

(52) What is COPD?
(A) Chronic outflow permeating disease.
(B) Chronic outflow pulmonary disease.
(C) Chronic obstructive percussive disease.
(D) Chronic obstructive pulmonary disease.

(53) What is the second part of the small intestine called?
(A) The duodenum.
(B) The jejunum.
(C) The ileum.
(D) All of the above.

(54) A patient's speech is slurred. What are some other signs a CNA should look out for?
(A) Weakness in any body part.
(B) Falls.
(C) Unconsciousness.
(D) All of the above.

(55) What are the major divisions of the nervous system?
(A) Central and peripheral.
(B) Frontal and posterior.
(C) Major and minor.
(D) Brain and spinal cord.

(56) What artery is used to measure the pulse?
(A) Axillary artery.
(B) Brachial artery.
(C) Ulnar artery.
(D) Radial artery.

(57) What are the characteristics to assess a pulse?
(A) Strength/volume.
(B) Rhythm.
(C) Rate.
(D) All of the above.

(58) What area should be focused on when respiration cycles are counted?
(A) Mouth.
(B) Nose.
(C) Chest.
(D) Stomach.

(59) What is not an accessory muscle of respiration?
(A) Sternocleidomastoid muscle.
(B) Pectoralis major.
(C) Pectoralis minor.
(D) Internal oblique.

(60) Which of the following is correct?
(A) The cuffs of gloves should never overlap the cuffs of a gown.
(B) The cuffs of gloves should overlap the cuffs of a gown.
(C) The cuffs of the gown should go over the cuffs of gloves.
(D) All of the above.

(61) After a procedure, a CNA should never:
(A) Remove their gown away from the body.
(B) Throw their gown on the floor.
(C) Wash their hands.
(D) Dispose of gloves in a designated waste container.

(62) Where should a gown be secured?
(A) At the neck and feet.
(B) At the waist and neck.
(C) At the waist and feet.
(D) At the neck, waist, and feet.

(63) A patient suffered a right-sided stroke and needs assistance with exercise. A CNA should not:
(A) Use gentle body movements.
(B) Move the joints through natural routes.
(C) Avoid over-extension.
(D) Use force on the affected side.

(64) How should a gown be removed from a patient with a right-sided weakness?
(A) From the right side.
(B) From the left side.
(C) From above.
(D) From anywhere.

(65) A CNA helps a patient dress. When he finishes, he should:
(A) Move to the next patient.
(B) Get another gown.
(C) Wash his hands.
(D) All of the above.

(66) What position must a client be in to eat?
(A) 50 to 80 degrees.
(B) Supine.
(C) 75 to 90 degrees.
(D) 180 degrees.

(67) What should be done before a patient is fed?
(A) Ask for the patient's name.
(B) Check for the patient's name card on the tray.
(C) Seek help.
(D) A and B.

(68) How should a CNA sit to feed a client?
(A) In front of the client.
(B) Beside the client.
(C) Behind the client.
(D) At the edge of the bed.

(69) What is an incorrect practice when feeding a client?
(A) Tell the client about the food and beverages on the food tray.
(B) Ask the client what they want to eat.
(C) Ask the client if they are ready for the next bite.
(D) Give the client beverages only after the meal.

(70) What position should the client be left in after a meal?

(A) 20 to 40 degrees.

(B) 180 degrees.

(C) 75 to 90 degrees.

(D) 360 degrees.

Test 4: Answers and Explanations

(1) (A) Delegation.

The staff nurse or RN delegates duties and responsibilities to CNAs. The duties may include measurement of patient vital signs, assisting patients with activities of daily living, etc.

(2) (B) Set a regular schedule for toileting to establish bladder control.

Bladder training is a method used to help patients regain control over their bladder function. It is usually used after surgery or when a patient has incontinence issues. A key role of a nursing assistant in this process is to assist the patient in setting and following a regular toileting schedule. This scheduled approach allows the bladder to gradually increase its holding capacity and control.

(3) (C) Safety.

The CNA failed to respond in time to attend to a patient in distress. This endangered the patient's need for safety.

(4) (C) Nonmaleficence.

Nonmaleficence encourages healthcare workers to do no harm to patients. This principle should not be taken literally. Sometimes, patients may be subjected to minor harm in the process of treatment. However, the benefits of such treatments must outweigh the risks of doing nothing.

(5) (B) Physical restraints should be released regularly.

Restraints are sometimes used to reduce the risk of harm or complications in an aggressive or overactive patient. Restraints include physical and chemical (drug) restraints. Physical restraints should be released regularly. Furthermore, restraints should not be used as punishments or to lessen the work of healthcare workers.

(6) (B) Greater than 7.0.

Diabetes mellitus is a chronic medical condition characterized by high blood sugar levels. It occurs as a result of absolute or relative insulin deficiency. There are two major types of diabetes mellitus. Type 1 is common in children. Type 2 is common in adults. Diagnosis is by a fasting blood sugar level of more than 7.0 mmol/L or a two-hour postprandial blood sugar level of more than 11.1 mmol/L.

(7) (A) Surgical bed.

Surgical beds are used when patients are brought to the ward from the operating room.

(8) (D) Nothing by mouth.

Nil per os means nothing by mouth. It is usually ordered for surgical patients shortly before and after abdominal procedures. It is also ordered for patients with intestinal obstructions and other such conditions.

(9) (A) It lasts longer than six months.

Chronic pain refers to pain that lasts longer than six months. It is a debilitating symptom that signifies an underlying chronic condition.

(10) (A) Computed tomography.

Stroke is a cerebrovascular disease that manifests with sudden-onset neurological deficit as a result of cerebral, spinal, or retinal hemorrhage or ischemia. It is diagnosed by a non-contrast CT scan of the brain or diffuse-weighted MRI.

(11) (A) Remind the patient her questions have already been answered.

When an individual with amnesia asks a question over and over, do not scold the person or point out you have already answered that question multiple times. Be empathetic and do not ignore the person.

(12) (C) Preschoolers.

Fear of the dark is a common fear in preschoolers (ages three to five years). Children in this age group are afraid of imaginary events. Some of the events may be what they see in movies. Adhere to the child's typical bedtime routine as much as possible.

(13) (A) Presbycusis.

Presbycusis is a common cause of sensorineural hearing loss that is associated with age. It occurs as a result of progressive damage to the cochlear hair cells. The other options in the list can cause deafness, but they are not usually related to age.

(14) (B) It is a chronic disease.

Asthma is a chronic, inflammatory, and hypersensitivity disease of the airway that causes reversible airway obstruction. Asthma can become complicated and cause respiratory failure if not properly treated. It can occur at any age, although it is often diagnosed in childhood. Treatment is airway relaxation and reduction of inflammation.

(15) (B) Chronic pain.

Chronic pain that lasts more than six months. It occurs mainly from chronic conditions, such as lumbar spondylosis, osteoarthritis, inflammatory muscle and bone diseases, and autoimmune diseases.

(16) (A) Edge of the bed.

Patients who are to be transferred to a wheelchair should be encouraged to move toward the edge of the bed. If patients cannot move, they should be supported to the edge of the bed and then transferred directly to the wheelchair. This helps to prevent injuries.

(17) (C) Maintain a routine, calm, and familiar environment.

It is important to establish and maintain a consistent routine and create a calm and familiar environment. This approach helps to minimize confusion and anxiety, which are common in individuals with Alzheimer's disease.

(18) (C) Proteins.

Proteins are an important food class that provides amino acids. These are mainly used in the production of body proteins such as muscles, cell components, structural molecules, enzymes, etc.

(19) (D) Immediately report your observation to the nurse.

A CNA should assess clients before the application of heat or cold and report any such observations to the nurse. Possible observations include a bluish skin color and poor sensation in the area where the heat or cold is to be applied.

(20) (B) Sit and talk with him for a while.

A CNA cannot create the care plan for a client, but they can report their observations to the nurse and then sit and talk with the man for a while.

(21) (C) Acceptance.

Acceptance is the period in which a person peacefully accepts their condition and its implications. The person may experience a sense of calm and be able to let go and move on. Acceptance does not mean that the person has given up hope. It simply means that the person has reached an emotional place that allows them to be at peace with the reality of the situation.

(22) (A) Generalized anxiety disorder.

Generalized anxiety disorder is characterized by excessive worry. Patients are often unable to carry out their normal daily activities due to persistent worry. This condition should be promptly evaluated and treated by a mental health specialist.

(23) (A) Therapeutic diet.

Therapeutic diets are tailored to meet the nutritional needs of each patient. For example, the DASH diet is recommended for patients with systemic hypertension to help lower blood pressure.

(24) (A) Urethral catheterization.

Patients with benign prostatic hyperplasia often develop urinary obstruction due to the enlarged prostate. Catheterization can be used to relieve the acute obstruction and achieve symptomatic relief. After the catheterization, pharmacological therapy can be used.

(25) (A) Cloudy and smelly urine.

Cloudy and smelly urine is often a sign of a UTI. When these signs are noticed, they should be reported to the charge nurse for further action.

(26) (D) Inform the nurse on duty.

Postoperative pain may arise from the surgical incision, or it could be an early sign of infection. When CNAs notice pain that is out of proportion to expectation, they should always inform the RN on duty.

(27) (A) Commercial straw holder.

A straw holder is useful for patients who cannot drink from a cup without spills. Such patients are usually elderly or have neuromuscular disorders such as amyotrophic lateral sclerosis. Multiple sclerosis or Parkinson's disease patients may also benefit from this utensil.

(28) (A) Wash their hands.

Hand hygiene is one of the most important health promotion strategies to prevent fecal-oral transmission of diseases.

(29) (A) Memory loss.

Amnesia is a term used to define memory loss. Dementia includes memory loss and impairment of thought, speech, and comprehension of the environment. Amnesia is seen in dementia, but not all patients with amnesia have dementia.

(30) (D) Delirium can be triggered by infections.

Delirium is a sudden reversible onset of decline in awareness and cognition. Infections are common causes of delirium, except in the elderly or in patients with neurodegenerative disorders.

(31) (B) Assist with gentle range-of-motion exercises as recommended.

For patients with arthritis, it's important to maintain joint function and mobility to the extent possible. You can assist with gentle range-of-motion exercises as recommended. These exercises help keep the joints flexible, reduce stiffness, and can alleviate pain.

(32) (A) Neurological disease.

Multiple sclerosis is a demyelinating neurological disease of the central nervous system that is characterized by plaque in the brain and spinal cord. This plaque causes hyperreflexia and movement problems. It may also cause autonomic problems.

(33) (D) Incentive spirometry.

Incentive spirometry can help postoperative patients prevent atelectasis. Atelectasis is the collapse of the lungs as a result of reduced inflation. It occurs commonly in postoperative patients because of reduced tidal activities due to pain.

(34) (D) Polycythemia.

Chronic kidney disease causes anemia (a reduced level of hematocrit). It does not cause polycythemia. Chronic kidney disease also causes leg swelling, facial puffiness, and hypertension. It may cause bleeding and neurological dysfunction in severe cases.

(35) (B) Inform the nurse.

If a CNA notices that a patient's nails are thick and unusually convex, the next best action is to inform the nurse. Thickened and convex nails could be indicative of a health issue, such as a fungal infection or other medical condition.

(36) (C) Help patients financially as the need arises.

CNAs must help patients adjust, build interactions with other individuals, and participate in daily routines. They educate patients on the importance of care, hygiene, relationships, and emotional support. This reduces anxiety and feelings of rejection, hopelessness, or dejection that patients might experience. CNAs are not in charge of patient finances.

(37) (D) Help the client connect with resources such as food banks, homeless shelters, and government assistance programs.

CNAs can help clients connect with resources such as food banks, homeless shelters, and government assistance programs.

(38) (B) Help the patient with prescribed exercises and proper body mechanics.

For a patient experiencing back pain, you should assist with exercises prescribed by a healthcare professional and encourage the use of proper body mechanics. This includes teaching and assisting with safe ways to bend, lift, and move that minimize stress on the back.

(39) (C) Death of spouse.

The death of a spouse is a major life change that can lead to loneliness and isolation. This is especially true if the spouse was the patient's primary social contact. Normal changes due to age, retirement, or a move to a new city are unlikely to be the reason for this client's loneliness.

(40) (C) The operating room.

Sterilization is most important in the operating room. This is because surgical procedures involve direct contact with sterile body areas or the vascular system, which makes them highly susceptible to infection.

(41) (B) Provide a quiet and dark environment to help alleviate symptoms.

A key supportive action you can take is to provide a quiet and dark environment. This can help reduce the intensity of migraine symptoms like light sensitivity and headache.

(42) (C) Turn the patient frequently.

A patient with a partial stroke might not be able to move the affected side of the body. Therefore, the patient needs to be turned every two hours so as not to develop bedsores.

(43) (B) Speaks.

A 70-year-old man with a fracture may have problems with movement and need help to take a bath or use the restroom. He could also have problems with eating. He at least needs someone to help him prepare the food. In the absence of any other comorbidity, the man should not have a problem with speech.

(44) (D) All of the above.

A stressed CNA cannot deliver optimal results. Therefore, there will be a drop in output, which might result in poor job performance. If the CNA falls ill or is not able to keep up, they might eventually be absent from work.

(45) (D) As a last resort to prevent harm to patients or others.

Restraints are only to be considered as a last resort to prevent harm to the patient or others. Restraints are not to be used as punishment, threats, or a means to silence someone.

(46) (A) Documented.

Whenever a drug is given to restrain a patient, appropriate documentation must be made for follow-up, in case of complications, and for medicolegal implications.

(47) (C) They're illegal.

This is incorrect. The use of restraints is not illegal. However, they must be used appropriately and only as a last resort.

(48) (D) Bartonella.

Bartonella is transmitted by fleas. Tuberculosis, chicken pox, and measles are all transmitted via airborne transmission.

(49) (C) Where two or more bones meet.

A joint is the location in the body where two or more bones meet. Joints are important components of the skeletal system and are responsible for providing flexibility and movement. They are the pivot points for motion and play a key role in activities such as walking, running, and grasping.

(50) (C) Bleeding.

A patient with a low platelet count (thrombocytopenia) is most at risk of bleeding. Platelets are a type of blood cell that play a crucial role in blood clotting. When platelet levels are low, the blood doesn't clot as effectively, which can cause increased bleeding. This can manifest as easy bruising, frequent nosebleeds, or bleeding gums. In more severe cases, it can cause internal bleeding, which can be life-threatening.

(51) (D) All of the above.

A patient with anemia has a low level of oxygen, which can put the patient at risk of falls, fainting, and breathlessness. A CNA must be on the lookout for any of these symptoms.

(52) (D) Chronic obstructive pulmonary disease.

COPD is a chronic respiratory disease that leads to restriction of airflow and problems with breathing. It comprises a group of diseases that include chronic bronchitis and emphysema.

(53) (B) The jejunum.

The second part of the small intestine is called the jejunum. The small intestine is divided into three sections: the duodenum, the jejunum, and the ileum. The duodenum is the first section, which is where the majority of chemical digestion occurs. The jejunum is the middle section, and it plays a major role in the absorption of nutrients from digested food. The ileum is the last part of the small intestine and is responsible for the absorption of vitamin B12 and bile salts.

(54) (D) All of the above.

This patient most likely had a stroke. Falls and unconsciousness are all symptoms that could happen again, so the CNA must be observant.

(55) (A) Central and peripheral.

The nervous system is divided into two major parts: the central nervous system (CNS) and the peripheral nervous system (PNS). The central nervous system consists of the brain and spinal cord. It acts as the control center for the body, which processes and sending out signals. The peripheral nervous system includes all the nerves that branch out from the brain and spinal cord and extend to other parts of the body (such as muscles, skin, and organs).

(56) (D) Radial artery.

The pulse is obtained from the radial artery, which passes through the lateral side of the wrist. It is a continuation of the brachial artery and supplies the forearm.

(57) (D) All of the above.

The strength assesses whether a pulse is weak or strong. The rhythm assesses whether a pulse is regular or irregular, and the rate assesses how many beats per minute. A normal pulse is strong/full volume, regular, and between 60 and 100 bpm.

(58) (C) Chest.

When counting respiration cycles, the focus should be on the chest. This is because the chest visibly rises and falls with each inhalation and exhalation, which makes it the most reliable and observable area for counting respirations.

(59) (D) Internal oblique.

The internal oblique muscle is located in the abdomen and forms part of the lateral abdominal wall. It is not an accessory muscle of respiration.

(60) (B) The cuffs of gloves should overlap the cuffs of the gown.

The cuffs of the gloves should always overlap the cuffs of the gown so that the gloves can be easily removed or changed. If the cuffs are under the gown, they will be difficult to remove without contamination.

(61) (B) Throw their gown on the floor.

After a procedure, a CNA should never throw their gown on the floor. Disposing of used personal protective equipment such as gowns on the floor is against infection control protocols and can contribute to the spread of contaminants and pathogens. Used gowns should be disposed of properly in designated waste containers or laundry hampers, depending on the facility's guidelines and the gown's material.

(62) (B) At the waist and neck.

A gown should be secured at the waist and neck. This ensures that the gown fits properly and provides adequate coverage and protection. Securing the gown at the neck keeps it in place around the upper body and shoulders, while tying it at the waist ensures that it stays wrapped around the body.

(63) (D) Use force on the affected side.

Applying force to the limbs on the side affected by a stroke can be harmful and cause injury, pain, or further impairment. Stroke patients often experience muscle weakness, paralysis, or a loss of control on the affected side. Gentle and careful handling is essential.

(64) (B) From the left side.

When removing a gown from a patient with right-sided weakness, it should be done from the left side (the patient's stronger side). This approach is important because it allows the patient to use their stronger side to assist in the removal process, which makes it easier and more comfortable for them.

(65) (C) Wash his hands.

After helping a patient with dressing, a CNA should wash his hands. Hand hygiene is an important step when preventing the spread of infections and maintaining a clean and safe environment for both the patient and the healthcare provider.

(66) (C) 75 to 90 degrees.

The client should be in an upright position to eat, which is usually between 75 to 90 degrees. This position is referred to as a high Fowler's position and helps prevent choking and facilitates swallowing.

(67) (D) A and B.

Before feeding a patient, you should confirm the patient's identity to ensure the right patient is receiving the correct meal. This can be done by asking for the patient's name and checking the patient's name card on the food tray.

(68) (B) Beside the client.

When feeding a client, you should sit beside them. This position allows you to maintain eye contact and interact more effectively with the client. It also facilitates easier assistance with eating and is more comfortable and respectful for both parties.

(69) (D) Give the client beverages only after the meal.

This is incorrect. Beverages should be provided to the client at least once during the meal, not only after.

(70) (C) 75 to 90 degrees.

The client should be left in a 75- to 90-degree position after meals. The client should not be bent over or lowered, which could increase the risk of aspiration.

Test 5: Questions

(1) A CNA should try to understand a patient's situation and general condition. This is known as:

(A) Pity.

(B) Empathy.

(C) Comprehension.

(D) Justice.

(2) Mrs. Johnson is a 45-year-old woman who lost her job as a storekeeper a year ago. Since then, she says things have not been the same. She was recently diagnosed with systemic hypertension. Which insurance program can Mrs. Johnson benefit from?

(A) Premium.

(B) Health maintenance organization.

(C) Medicaid.

(D) Medicare.

(3) Which term describes the verbal exchange of medical information between members of the healthcare team?

(A) Relay.

(B) Report.

(C) Document.

(D) Consult.

(4) A nurse has just delegated a CNA to monitor the blood pressure of a patient with severe hypertension every two hours. When CNA Nicole gets to the patient, he declines her request to measure his blood pressure. What principle of medical ethics will the CNA break if she goes ahead and measures the patient's blood pressure anyway?

(A) Autonomy.

(B) Integrity.

(C) Nonmaleficence.

(D) Justice.

(5) Which of the following increases the risk of falls?

(A) Neurological disease.

(B) Sex.

(C) Body mass index.

(D) Exercise level.

(6) How should you respond when caring for a patient experiencing delirium?
(A) Engage in complex conversations to stimulate the patient's brain.
(B) Restrict all visitors to prevent overstimulation.
(C) Provide a calm and reassuring presence.
(D) Encourage the patient to sleep as little as possible.

(7) A 66-year-old patient is admitted for treatment of a diabetic emergency. Which of the following will help to protect the patient's privacy on the ward?
(A) Privacy board.
(B) Privacy sheets.
(C) Privacy curtains.
(D) Bed cradle.

(8) Mr. Joe is a 68-year-old man admitted to the medical ward on account of diabetic complications. He develops burning with urination and fever on admission. Which investigation can help point to the diagnosis?
(A) Urine protein.
(B) Urine glucose.
(C) Urine microscopy and culture.
(D) Urine specific gravity.

(9) How should you assist a patient experiencing tinnitus?
(A) Provide loud music to mask the tinnitus sounds.
(B) Engage in shouting conversations to be heard over the tinnitus.
(C) Ensure a quiet and calm environment to reduce irritation from tinnitus.
(D) Advise the patient to ignore the sounds as they are not real.

(10) What is an important aspect of care for a patient with an ulcer?
(A) Encourage the patient to eat spicy foods to build tolerance.
(B) Regularly reposition the patient to prevent pressure ulcers.
(C) Apply tight bandages to restrict movement of the affected area.
(D) Ignore the ulcer as it is self-healing.

(11) Mr. Allen, a 76-year-old man who worked for 40 years as a radio broadcaster, is brought to the hospital due to an inability to understand communication in both written and spoken form. What is this condition known as?

(A) Expressive aphasia.

(B) Receptive aphasia.

(C) Agnosia.

(D) Amnesia.

(12) What is not one way to ensure the safety of an infant?

(A) Be sure to lock the wheels of the stroller.

(B) Keep the rails of the crib up at all times.

(C) Never leave the infant unattended.

(D) Don't allow the infant to have any toys.

(13) Which device is used to improve hearing in patients with an auditory impairment?

(A) Earphones.

(B) Headphones.

(C) Hearing aids.

(D) Speakers.

(14) An elderly female with acute asthma exacerbation should be helped to:

(A) Locate an oxygen cylinder.

(B) Locate her inhaler.

(C) Drink some water.

(D) Locate oral steroids.

(15) A 34-year-old woman is rushed to the clinic with features suggestive of heart failure. The senior nurse instructs the CNA to put the patient in a low Fowler's position. This position is:

(A) Supine.

(B) Prone.

(C) With the head of the bed raised 30 degrees.

(D) With the foot of the bed raised 30 degrees.

(16) Which of the following positions are not correctly matched?
(A) Sim's – a patient lies on his side.
(B) Fowler's – a patient's head is raised.
(C) Supine – a patient lies on his stomach.
(D) Low Fowler's – a patient's head is raised.

(17) What is a possible complication of poor perineal hygiene?
(A) Urinary tract infection.
(B) Ectopic pregnancy.
(C) Fibroids.
(D) Cellulitis.

(18) A 35-year-old woman's body mass index is 41 kg/m2. Which of the following is not a risk factor for her weight?
(A) Activity level.
(B) Diet.
(C) Alcohol consumption.
(D) Sex.

(19) To promote sleep and rest, a patient should not:
(A) Create a restful environment.
(B) Avoid physical activities during the day.
(C) Have a familiar bedtime routine.
(D) Nap during the day.

(20) All of the following are the needs of a dying person except:
(A) Dignity.
(B) Lies.
(C) Preparation for death.
(D) Hygiene.

(21) A person and those close to the person may experience all of the following during the end-of-life period except:
(A) Acceptance.
(B) Hope.
(C) Fear.
(D) Indifference.

(22) A 50-year-old woman is admitted with auditory hallucinations and delusions. The symptoms are best classified as:

(A) Psychotic.

(B) Neurotic.

(C) Anxiety.

(D) Phobia.

(23) A carbohydrate-controlled diet is ordered for people with:

(A) Diabetes.

(B) Hypertension.

(C) Heart failure.

(D) Dyslipidemia.

(24) Which of the following best helps to promote elimination?

(A) Food low in fiber.

(B) Reminders to use the restroom.

(C) Consumption of less water.

(D) A regular elimination pattern.

(25) Which test can be used to diagnose diabetes?

(A) Urinalysis.

(B) Urine microscopy.

(C) Urine culture.

(D) Fasting blood sugar.

(26) Rheumatoid arthritis causes:

(A) Acute pain.

(B) Chronic pain.

(C) Subacute pain.

(D) Acute or chronic pain.

(27) A 55-year-old patient with Parkinson's disease cannot keep food on the spoon/fork because of tremors. Which of the following may benefit this patient?

(A) A swivel fork or spoon.

(B) A long spoon.

(C) A short spoon.

(D) A metallic spoon.

(28) CNAs help provide patients with oral, facial, and hair care. This is referred to as:
(A) Cleanliness.
(B) Hygiene.
(C) Grooming.
(D) Spa day.

(29) A 66-year-old woman with dementia is noticed to have memory loss. In addition, she also has a speech impairment. The speech impairment is referred to as:
(A) Aphasia.
(B) Apraxia.
(C) Agnosia.
(D) Amnesia.

(30) What is the main purpose of using a pulse oximeter in patient care?
(A) To measure the patient's body temperature.
(B) To assess the patient's cognitive abilities.
(C) To determine the oxygen saturation level in the patient's blood.
(D) To calculate the patient's blood pressure.

(31) Which of the following measures can help a patient with poor circulation?
(A) Elevation of arms and feet.
(B) Cooling.
(C) Rest.
(D) Diet.

(32) All of the following patients need help with mobility, except a/an:
(A) Stroke patient.
(B) Spinal cord injury patient.
(C) Lower limb fracture patient.
(D) Amnesia patient.

(33) Which measurement is most important in the management of patients with COPD?
(A) Pulse oximetry.
(B) Ankle-brachial index.
(C) Body mass index.
(D) Waist-hip ratio.

(34) Which of the following refers to a disease characterized by abnormal growth of cells that crowd other normal cells?

(A) Swelling.

(B) Cancer.

(C) Pimples.

(D) Boil.

(35) What is an important aspect of care for a patient with kidney disease?

(A) Restricting all fluids to reduce kidney workload.

(B) Providing high-sodium foods to improve kidney function.

(C) Monitoring and recording fluid intake and output accurately.

(D) Encouraging the consumption of alcohol to stimulate the kidneys.

(36) Which of the following is important when it comes to patient privacy?

(A) The CNA should monitor every activity of the client.

(B) The CNA should assign a relative to monitor every activity of the client.

(C) The CNA should ignore patient privacy to provide adequate care.

(D) The CNA should ensure that patients have private spaces where they can relax.

(37) A 65-year-old woman doesn't feel safe. How can a CNA help?

(A) Report the situation to the woman's family members.

(B) Give the woman a gun for her safety.

(C) Tell the woman not to leave her home.

(D) Create a safe and supportive environment for the woman and help her develop coping mechanisms for stress and anxiety.

(38) Alterations in cognitive function can lead to all of the following except:

(A) Poor judgment.

(B) Incontinence.

(C) Self-harm.

(D) Happiness.

(39) An 80-year-old man presents to the clinic with his son. He says his children constantly criticize him and order him around. What is the most likely reason for this patient's relationship changes?

(A) Normal changes due to aging.

(B) Retirement.

(C) Health problems.

(D) Role reversal.

(40) How is Hepatitis B mostly transmitted to healthcare workers?

(A) Sexual intercourse.

(B) Fecal-oral route.

(C) Infected needles.

(D) All of the above.

(41) Which of the following is true about the preparation of formalin?

(A) It should be labeled appropriately.

(B) People should not eat or drink around the chemical.

(C) People should not put their mouths on the pipette.

(D) All of the above.

(42) A diabetic patient complains of an inability to feel her shoes. What advice should a CNA offer?

(A) Always walk around barefoot.

(B) Do not walk around barefoot.

(C) The feeling will subside.

(D) It's nothing to worry about.

(43) A 65-year-old Caucasian woman is diagnosed with osteoporosis. What is the most likely risk factor in this patient?

(A) Age.

(B) Sex.

(C) Race.

(D) Both A and B.

(44) How often should an unconscious patient be turned to avoid bedsores?
(A) Every hour.
(B) Every two hours.
(C) Every three hours.
(D) Every four hours.

(45) Which class of drug is not used to restrain patients?
(A) Antipsychotics.
(B) Antiemetics.
(C) Sedatives.
(D) Antidepressants.

(46) What is not a risk factor for elopement?
(A) Lack of close monitoring by health professionals.
(B) Medical history of wandering.
(C) Neurological disorders.
(D) Middle age.

(47) If a CNA wants to use restraints on a patient, she should tell the patient's relatives:
(A) The benefits of restraints.
(B) The side effects of restraints.
(C) The alternatives to restraints.
(D) All of the above.

(48) Which of the following diseases and vectors are correctly matched?
(A) Malaria – dirofilaria spp.
(B) Lyme disease – microspora.
(C) Plague – fleas.
(D) Heartworm disease – malaria.

(49) What advice should a CNA give a 67-year-old female patient recently diagnosed with osteoporosis?
(A) Avoid calcium.
(B) Use handrails to prevent falls.
(C) Limit the use of glasses.
(D) Develop a personal exercise routine.

(50) A patient presents with leukocytopenia. What is the patient most likely to experience?
(A) Swollen gums.
(B) Recurrent infections.
(C) Anemia.
(D) All of the above.

(51) Which of the following is not part of the respiratory system?
(A) The nose.
(B) The sinuses.
(C) The larynx.
(D) The sternocleidomastoid.

(52) What are the two major forms of COPD?
(A) Asthma and allergies.
(B) Asthma and tuberculosis.
(C) Emphysema and asthma.
(D) Chronic bronchitis and emphysema.

(53) What is a common injury in the mucosa of the duodenum called?
(A) An ulcer.
(B) Cancer.
(C) A malignant transformation.
(D) Leukemia.

(54) What are the things a CNA should pay special attention to in an unconscious patient?
(A) Oral hygiene.
(B) Bedsores.
(C) Position.
(D) All of the above.

(55) If an unconscious patient begins to show signs of consciousness, a CNA should:
(A) Start medications.
(B) Inform the nurse immediately.
(C) Speak to the patient.
(D) All of the above.

(56) What is an important action when caring for a patient with respiratory problems?
(A) Encourage the patient to hold their breath for long periods.
(B) Keep the patient in a flat, supine position at all times.
(C) Assist with and promote effective deep breathing exercises.
(D) Advise the patient to smoke lightly to strengthen the lungs.

(57) When a patient is given a bed bath, it is unnecessary for the CNA to:
(A) Check the water temperature for safety.
(B) Put on clean gloves.
(C) Ask the client to verify their comfort with the water temperature.
(D) Ask the patient what body part they want to start the bed bath from.

(58) Which of the following is incorrect when a patient is given a bath?
(A) The same washcloth can be used throughout.
(B) Soap and water should be applied to the washcloth.
(C) Soap should not be used when a patient's eyes are cleaned.
(D) A patient's privacy must be ensured.

(59) Before a bedpan is handled, a CNA must:
(A) Wear clean gloves.
(B) Rinse the bedpan.
(C) Measure the urine in the bedpan.
(D) All of the above.

(60) In which of the following conditions is the measurement of urine output nonnegotiable?
(A) Malaria.
(B) Heart failure.
(C) Acute kidney injury.
(D) Rhinosinusitis.

(61) In what position should urine be measured in the container?
(A) From above.
(B) At eye level.
(C) From below.
(D) Any position is fine.

(62) Which precautions should a CNA take before an ambulatory client is weighed?
(A) Do an X-ray.
(B) Ensure the client wears footwear.
(C) Ensure that the scale is set to zero.
(D) All of the above.

(63) Where should clients stand when they are weighed?
(A) At the center of the scale.
(B) At the end of the scale.
(C) On one leg at the right side of the scale.
(D) Anywhere as long as the scale indicator moves.

(64) What is the usual unit of measurement of weight?
(A) Lbs/Kg.
(B) Cm/M.
(C) Km/m.
(D) Newtons.

(65) How many times should flexion/extension be carried out when a modified passive range of motion is carried out on a patient's leg?
(A) Once.
(B) Twice.
(C) Thrice.
(D) Four times.

(66) What should be done if a client verbalizes pain?
(A) Stop the movement for a few seconds and continue.
(B) Stop the movement completely.
(C) Ignore the patient, as the pain will subside.
(D) Reassure the patient.

(67) In plantar flexion, what happens to the toes?
(A) They point up.
(B) They point down.
(C) They point sideways.
(D) They point straight.

(68) When a CNA performs a PROM for the right shoulder, the arm should be supported:
(A) At the forearm.
(B) At the elbow.
(C) At the wrist.
(D) Both B and C.

(69) What is an important post-operative care task to perform for a patient who has undergone surgery?
(A) Encourage the patient to remain immobile to promote healing.
(B) Frequently change the patient's position to prevent bedsores.
(C) Immediately remove all surgical dressings to inspect the wound.
(D) Instruct the patient to lift heavy objects as a form of physical therapy.

(70) What movements are performed in a PROM for the shoulder?
(A) Extension.
(B) Abduction.
(C) Flexion.
(D) All of the above.

Test 5: Answers and Explanations

(1) (B) Empathy.

Empathy is the attempt to understand patients' concerns and points of view. It involves consideration of patients' spiritual, physical, and psychosocial contexts. Empathy is a quality that every CNA is required to possess in order to perform their role effectively.

(2) (C) Medicaid.

Medicaid is a federal program that provides health coverage for financially incapacitated members of society. This patient, who lost her job and has been unable to afford insurance coverage, is a potential candidate for Medicaid.

(3) (B) Report.

CNAs are delegated to carry out specific tasks. If they find a deviation from the norm, they have a duty to report it to an RN.

(4) (A) Autonomy.

If Nicole takes the patient's blood pressure in spite of his refusal, she will violate the principle of patient autonomy. Autonomy is a core principle of medical ethics that protects the rights of patients to make decisions about their health.

(5) (A) Neurological disease.

A patient with a history of neurological disease is at risk of falls. This is because neurological disease affects a patient's balance, gait, and posture as a result of weakness in muscle groups due to muscle paralysis.

(6) (C) Provide a calm and reassuring presence.

When caring for a patient experiencing delirium, it is important to provide a calm and reassuring presence. This means speaking to the patient in a gentle, soothing manner, ensuring the environment is safe and quiet, and reducing factors that might contribute to confusion or agitation.

(7) (C) Privacy curtains.

Curtains are used to provide privacy for patients in a shared admission room or a big ward with multiple patients. The privacy curtains are used when patients are examined, or procedures are performed.

(8) (C) Urine microscopy and culture.

Urine microscopy and culture are investigations used to diagnose UTIs. They involve direct visualization of a urine specimen under the microscope, followed by culture and examination. UTIs present with urinary frequency, urgency, and dysuria.

(9) (C) Ensure a quiet and calm environment to reduce irritation from tinnitus.

Tinnitus is characterized by ringing or other noises in one or both ears that are not caused by an external sound. A nurse aide should aim to create a quiet and calm environment.

(10) (B) Regularly reposition the patient to prevent pressure ulcers.

For patients who are bedridden or have limited mobility, regularly reposition them to prevent the development of pressure ulcers (bedsores). This means that the patient's position should be changed every few hours to alleviate pressure on areas of the body that are at risk, such as the back, hips, and heels.

(11) (B) Receptive aphasia.

Aphasia refers to problems with communication due to damage to the brain or disease, and receptive aphasia refers to an inability to understand both spoken and written communication. Expressive aphasia refers to an inability to use language to express one's thoughts. Agnosia is the inability to use the five senses to recognize familiar things. Amnesia is the term used to describe memory loss.

(12) (D) Don't allow the infant to have any toys.

Use only age-appropriate toys with an infant. Remember that infants like to put everything in their mouths. Be sure that toys have no small parts that can be swallowed.

(13) (C) Hearing aids.

Hearing aids are devices that are used to improve hearing in patients. Hearing impairment can result from the impairment of conduction of sound (conductive hearing loss). It may also occur from damage to nerve cells or the sensory organs of the ear (sensorineural hearing loss).

(14) (B) Locate her inhaler.

When patients develop acute exacerbation of asthma, they often have worsening of their usual symptoms. Such patients should be helped to use their inhalers and then get emergency medical attention to establish normal respiratory function. Untreated severe asthma exacerbation can result in respiratory failure and death.

(15) (C) With the head of the bed raised 30 degrees.

The Low Fowler's position is used for some specific patients. The foot of the bed is raised 30 degrees. This position is used for patients with cardiac diseases such as congestive cardiac failure to facilitate easy relief of lung congestion.

(16) (C) Supine – a patient lies on his stomach.

The supine position does not involve a patient lying on their stomach. Rather, it is when a patient lies on their back and faces upwards. This is a fundamental position in medical care for various examinations and procedures. The other positions listed are correctly matched. Sim's position is where the patient lies on their side, the lower arm is behind the back and the upper thigh is flexed. In Fowler's position, the patient's head and upper body are raised at a 45- to 60-degree angle, and Low Fowler's position is a variation where the head and upper body are raised at a lower angle, between 15 and 30 degrees.

(17) (A) Urinary tract infections.

Poor perineal hygiene increases the risk of infections, especially in patients at assisted living facilities. Patients who need help with perineal hygiene should receive prompt help to reduce the risk of infections.

(18) (D) Sex.

This patient with a 41 kg/m2 body mass index is morbidly obese. Morbid obesity is associated with cardiovascular, emotional, and physical complications. Risk factors for obesity include a sedentary lifestyle, poor diet, lack of exercise, alcohol consumption, etc. Sex is not a risk factor.

(19) (B) Avoid physical activities during the day.

Physical activities during the day are one of the best strategies to promote both rest and sleep.

(20) (B) Lies.

The needs of a dying person include being told the truth about their condition. Other needs may include preparation of the person for death, hygiene, providing company for the patient, ensuring the person is free of physical discomfort and pain, and listening.

(21) (D) Indifference.

Indifference is not part of the common emotions expressed by dying people or those close to them. Examples of emotions expressed include hope, anger, sadness, grief, and acceptance.

(22) (A) Psychotic.

Psychotic symptoms are delusions, hallucinations, and disorganized thinking. Delusions are unusual beliefs that are not in tandem with reality. Hallucinations are experiences that are not real, but patients think they are. Both delusions and hallucinations are prominent in psychotic disorders like schizophrenia.

(23) (A) Diabetes.

Because people with diabetes mellitus have problems with insulin regulation of blood sugar, a carbohydrate-controlled diet is often recommended for them. Because the diet is low in sugar, this helps to improve sugar control.

(24) (D) A regular elimination pattern.

A regular elimination pattern helps to promote bowel hygiene. This helps to prevent constipation.

(25) (D) Fasting blood sugar.

Fasting blood sugar is a common investigation that is ordered after at least eight hours of fasting. It is used to diagnose diabetes mellitus. A value above 7 mmol/l is usually diagnostic. Apart from fasting blood sugar, postprandial or random blood sugar can also be used to diagnose diabetes.

(26) (B) Chronic pain.

Rheumatoid arthritis is a chronic inflammatory disorder that is characterized by joint destruction, early morning stiffness, and joint pain. It can be associated with other autoimmune diseases like vitiligo, type 1 diabetes mellitus, or systemic lupus erythematous. Rheumatoid arthritis causes chronic pain.

(27) (A) A swivel fork or spoon.

Some patients can't keep food on the spoon because of unsteadiness or tremors. Such patients will benefit from a swivel fork or spoon, which is designed to hold food in place.

(28) (C) Grooming.

Well-groomed patients have their hair combed, are dressed appropriately, and maintain good oral hygiene.

(29) (A) Aphasia.

Aphasia is speech impairment that is associated with dementia and other neurodegenerative diseases.

(30) (C) To determine the oxygen saturation level in the patient's blood.

Pulse oximetry is a non-invasive method used to measure the oxygen saturation level, or the amount of oxygen carried in the blood. This is an important vital sign that helps to assess how well oxygen is being delivered to parts of the patient's body furthest from the heart, such as the arms and legs.

(31) (A) Elevation of arms and feet.

Patients with poor circulation should be advised to elevate their arms and feet to improve circulation.

(32) (D) Amnesia patient.

Amnesia is a loss of memory. It can be anterograde or retrograde. Anterograde amnesia results in a failure to form new memories. Retrograde amnesia causes the loss of past memories. Amnesia is not a movement disorder and does not cause weakness. It does not require help with mobility.

(33) (A) Pulse oximetry.

In patients with COPD, regular pulse oximetry checks are important to monitor treatment progress. This is also used to determine the modality of airway management. Severe hypoxia is usually managed differently from mild hypoxia.

(34) (B) Cancer.

Cancer is characterized by the abnormal growth of cells. The cells eventually cause necrosis, pain, bleeding, weight loss, and other symptoms based on the type of cancer.

(35) (C) Monitoring and recording fluid intake and output accurately.

It's important to carefully monitor and record the fluid intake and output. This is because the kidneys may not be able to regulate fluid balance effectively, which can cause complications such as fluid overload or dehydration.

(36) (D) The CNA should ensure that patients have private spaces where they can relax.

CNAs should ensure that patients have private spaces where they can relax when needed. Also, bathrooms should not be exposed. This is a way to promote respect for patients' privacy during personal care routines and when they receive visitors.

(37) (D) Create a safe and supportive environment for the woman and help her develop coping mechanisms for stress and anxiety.

CNAs can create a safe and supportive environment for the client in the therapy room. They can also help the client develop mechanisms to deal with stress and anxiety.

(38) (D) Happiness.

Alteration in cognitive functions can also lead to poor judgment, incontinence, self-harm, and isolation among the elderly. Hence, care should be provided with compassion and respect for dignity so that patients can express themselves without guilt or shame.

(39) (D) Role reversal.

As people age, it is normal for their roles in relationships to change. For example, parents may become more dependent on their children. This can lead to conflict and resentment, especially if the children are not prepared for this change.

(40) (C) Infected needles.

Infected needles are the most common way diseases like hepatitis B and HIV are transmitted to healthcare workers.

(41) (D) All of the above.

All formalin bottles and containers should be labeled appropriately. People should not eat or drink during the formalin preparation to minimize the risk of accidental ingestion. CNAs should not put the pipette in their mouth for any reason.

(42) (B) Do not walk around barefoot.

Due to the neuropathy associated with the condition, people with diabetes might not be able to feel sensations, even when they have injuries. As a result, patients with diabetes should not walk around barefoot.

(43) (D) Both A and B.

Age is a major risk factor for osteoporosis. As women age, their bones get more brittle because they no longer produce estrogen. Another risk factor is gender. Osteoporosis is more common in women than men.

(44) (B) Every two hours.

An unconscious patient should be turned every two hours to prevent the development of bedsores (also known as pressure ulcers). Bedsores are injuries to the skin and underlying tissue that result from prolonged pressure on the skin. They often develop on skin that covers bony areas of the body, such as the heels, ankles, hips, and the tailbone. Regularly turning or repositioning a patient helps to redistribute pressure and promote blood circulation, which reduces the risk of pressure ulcer formation.

(45) (B) Antiemetics.

Antiemetics are drugs given to stop vomiting, not restrain patients. All other classes of drugs have sedating effects and can be used to restrain patients when needed as a last resort.

(46) (D) Middle age.

Middle age is not generally considered a risk factor for elopement, especially in the context of healthcare settings or among individuals with cognitive impairments. Elopement refers to a patient or resident who leaves a facility unsupervised and potentially places themselves in danger.

(47) (D) All of the above.

CNAs are required to explain the importance, benefits, side effects, and alternatives of restraints to the relatives of patients and obtain informed consent if the patient is unable to communicate.

(48) (C) Plague – fleas.

The plague is correctly matched with fleas as its vector. Plague is a disease caused by the bacterium Yersinia pestis, which can be transmitted to humans through the bite of infected fleas. These fleas live on wild rodents but can infect humans and domestic animals. The other pairs are incorrectly matched.

(49) (B) Use handrails to prevent falls.

Falls are very common in this age group, and when there is a fall, there is an increased tendency for fractures due to osteoporosis. Using handrails will reduce the risk of falls in this patient.

(50) (B) Recurrent infections.

Leukocytopenia is a condition in which a patient has a low number of white blood cells. When there are low white blood cells, the patient is prone to infection.

(51) (D) The sternocleidomastoid.

The sternocleidomastoid is not part of the respiratory system. It is a muscle in the neck that plays a role in head movement and posture. The other options listed – the nose, the sinuses, and the larynx – are all components of the respiratory system. The nose is involved in the inhalation and filtration of air, the sinuses help regulate the temperature and humidity of inhaled air, and the larynx, or voice box, is vital for phonation and provides an air passage to the lungs.

(52) (D) Chronic bronchitis and emphysema.

COPD is a chronic respiratory disease that leads to the restriction of airflow and problems with breathing. It comprises a group of diseases that include chronic bronchitis and emphysema.

(53) (A) An ulcer.

A common injury in the mucosa of the duodenum is called an ulcer, or specifically a duodenal ulcer. This type of ulcer is a sore that develops on the lining of the duodenum, which is the first part of the small intestine. Duodenal ulcers are often caused by an infection with the bacterium Helicobacter pylori or by the prolonged use of nonsteroidal anti-inflammatory drugs (NSAIDs).

(54) (D) All of the above.

The CNA must pay attention to oral hygiene, frequently turn the patient to prevent bedsores, and position the person appropriately for different activities.

(55) (B) Inform the nurse immediately.

If an unconscious patient begins to show signs of regaining consciousness, a CNA should inform the nurse immediately. The nurse can then assess the patient's condition and determine the appropriate next steps for care.

(56) Assist with and promote effective deep breathing exercises.

These exercises can help improve lung function, clear airways, and enhance oxygenation, which is critical for individuals with respiratory difficulties.

(57) (D) Ask the patient what body part they want to start the bed bath from.

There are standard protocols for giving baths. The role of the CNA is to explain to the patient what they are about to do, not ask them what to do.

(58) (A) The same washcloth can be used throughout.

This is incorrect. When the body of a client is cleaned, a CNA should use at least two washcloths—one wet washcloth to clean the patient and another dry washcloth for use after the bath to dry the patient.

(59) (A) Wear clean gloves.

Before handling a bedpan, a CNA must wear clean gloves. This practice is important for infection control and personal protection. Wearing gloves helps prevent the spread of germs and protects the CNA from coming into contact with bodily fluids, which is especially important when dealing with waste elimination tools like bedpans.

(60) (C) Acute kidney injury.

Urine output is a general measure of a patient's health that should always be taken, and its measurement is nonnegotiable in acute kidney injury.

(61) (B) At eye level.

For the measurement of urine, a graded measuring container is usually used. The container should be placed on a flat surface, and measurements should be taken at eye level.

(62) (C) Ensure that the scale is set to zero.

When you want to measure the weight of an ambulatory client, ensure that the weight of the scale is set to zero to obtain correct values.

(63) (A) At the center of the scale.

When being weighed, clients should stand at the center of the scale. This positioning ensures the most accurate and balanced measurement of their weight. Standing in the center allows the weight to be evenly distributed on the scale, which means the reading will be precise.

(64) (A) Lbs/Kg.

The usual units of measurement for weight are pounds (lbs) and kilograms (Kg). In the United States, pounds are commonly used, while kilograms are the standard unit of weight in the metric system and are widely used internationally. Both lbs and Kg are measures of mass, and represent the weight of an object or person.

(65) (C) Thrice.

When performing modified passive range of motion exercises on a patient's leg, each movement, such as flexion (bending) and extension (straightening), should be carried out three times. This repetition is important for effectively maintaining or improving joint function and mobility. It allows the muscles and joints to be adequately stretched and moved, which helps to preserve flexibility and reduce stiffness.

(66) (B) Stop the movement completely.

If a client verbalizes pain during a movement or activity, the movement should be stopped completely. Continuing the movement, even after pausing could exacerbate the pain or cause further injury. It is important to acknowledge the client's discomfort and not ignore it, as this could mean neglecting a potentially serious issue.

(67) (B) They point down.

In plantar flexion, the toes point downwards. This movement occurs when the angle between the foot and the leg decreases, as is seen when pressing down on a gas pedal or standing on tiptoes. Plantar flexion is the opposite of dorsiflexion, where the toes point upwards towards the shin. Pointing the toes sideways or straight does not describe plantar flexion. The key characteristic of plantar flexion is the downward movement of the toes and the foot, which engages the muscles in the back of the lower leg.

(68) (D) Both B and C.

When a CNA performs Passive Range of Motion (PROM) exercises for the right shoulder, it is important to support the arm at both the elbow and the wrist. This dual support ensures stability and safety during the exercise. Supporting at the elbow helps to maintain proper alignment of the arm and shoulder, while supporting at the wrist helps control the movement and protect the joints and muscles from strain or injury.

(69) Frequently change the patient's position to prevent bedsores.

After surgery, it's important for a patient's recovery to prevent the development of bedsores, especially if their mobility is limited. A nurse aide frequently helps the patient change positions. This not only helps to alleviate pressure on certain areas of the body but also promotes circulation, which is essential for healing.

(70) (D) All of the above.

PROM movements at the shoulder include flexion/extension and abduction/adduction.

Test 6: Questions

(1) All of the following are duties CNAs have to their patients, except:

(A) Protection of personal dignity.

(B) Protection of privacy.

(C) Patient safety.

(D) Provision of intravenous access.

(2) Which regulatory bodies provide guidelines to protect healthcare workers from hazards?

(A) Health Maintenance Act.

(B) Occupational Safety and Health Administration.

(C) Occupational Regulation.

(D) Labor Act.

(3) Why might a nurse aide assist a patient in using a spirometer?

(A) To improve the patient's singing abilities.

(B) To enhance lung function after surgery or during lung illness.

(C) To measure the patient's blood pressure.

(D) For entertainment purposes.

(4) A staff nurse discusses the importance of infection prevention and control in patient management. She mentions a few methods of infection prevention. Which of the following is the most important method?

(A) Immunization.

(B) Handwashing.

(C) PPE.

(D) Routine screening.

(5) A 35-year-old man convulses at home. He is a known patient of the neurology unit, where he is being managed for a seizure disorder. Which measure is most appropriate for a relative to take at home to help the patient?

(A) Pour water on the patient.

(B) Put objects in the patient's mouth to prevent his teeth from clenching.

(C) Help the patient sit down comfortably.

(D) Lay the patient in the left lateral position and call 911.

(6) Which symptoms are seen in a patient with myocardial infarction?
(A) Dyspnea, orthopnea, swollen legs.
(B) Severe central chest pain that radiates to the arms, diaphoresis.
(C) Weakness, nausea, vomiting.
(D) Fast breathing, fever, cough.

(7) An immobile patient who is expected to spend weeks on the ward must be turned regularly in bed. This action prevents:
(A) Bedsores.
(B) Stroke.
(C) Heart failure.
(D) Arthritis.

(8) Mid-stream urine collection means:
(A) The patient's total daily urine output.
(B) The patient's early morning urine.
(C) Half of the patient's total daily urine.
(D) The patient starts the urine stream, stops, then restarts and collects the sample.

(9) A woman has just been admitted to a healthcare facility. How best should a CNA initiate communication with the patient to foster a therapeutic alliance?
(A) Assume the patient's pronouns.
(B) Refer to the patient by her ID number.
(C) Greet the patient and ask how she would like to be addressed.
(D) Do not greet the patient until she introduces herself.

(10) Which investigations can be used to diagnose myocardial infarction?
(A) Chest X-ray.
(B) Heart scan.
(C) Electrocardiogram.
(D) Fasting blood sugar.

(11) Mr. James is brought to the hospital with his heart and breathing stopped. He signed a DNR-CC order. Which of the following interventions should not be done?

(A) Administration of oxygen.

(B) Administration of pain relief.

(C) Initiation of cardiopulmonary resuscitation.

(D) Initiation of supportive care.

(12) A 15-year-old girl who has been involved in an accident is under a CNA's care. What should the CNA do to help this patient?

(A) Encourage her imagination.

(B) Provide for the girl's privacy.

(C) Help the girl complete tasks.

(D) Use simple terms to interact with the girl.

(13) An 80-year-old patient with osteoarthritis treated with over-the-counter painkillers develops ringing in her ear. What is the most likely diagnosis?

(A) Tinnitus.

(B) Deafness.

(C) Hearing loss.

(D) Presbycusis.

(14) What is not a symptom of acute asthma exacerbation?

(A) Cough.

(B) Dyspnea.

(C) Swollen legs.

(D) Wheezing.

(15) A 65-year-old patient is to be moved from the ward to the radiology unit for a brain MRI. Which factor should be considered when the patient is moved?

(A) Age.

(B) Gender.

(C) Mobility.

(D) The investigation to be done.

(16) Which equipment may be used to facilitate adequate body positioning while a patient lies in the lateral position?
(A) Bed cradle.
(B) Sheets.
(C) Positioning aids.
(D) Pneumatic bed.

(17) What is a possible complication of poor oral care?
(A) Diabetes.
(B) Hypertension.
(C) Dental caries.
(D) HIV.

(18) A 66-year-old woman was diagnosed with type 2 diabetes mellitus a year ago but has not needed any medication since then as her blood sugar has been well controlled. Which of the following is a likely explanation for her blood sugar control?
(A) Diet.
(B) Local herbs.
(C) Increased salt intake.
(D) Regular sleep.

(19) All of the following are examples of chronic pain except:
(A) Cancer pain.
(B) Osteoarthritis pain.
(C) Osteoporotic pain.
(D) Pain from a fall.

(20) Mrs. Goodluck, a 46-year-old woman, was just told that she has cancer. She says it is impossible because her religion and culture forbid it. Which of the following is Mrs. Goodluck expressing?
(A) Hope.
(B) Fear.
(C) Denial.
(D) Anger.

(21) Some relatives ask a CNA what they can do to help their dying sister. The family members of a dying person should be:

(A) Encouraged to speak about their needs and feelings.

(B) Encouraged to leave the dying person alone.

(C) Discouraged from participation in the care of the dying person.

(D) Discouraged from expressing their feelings.

(22) Which of the following is a symptom of severe depression?

(A) Denial.

(B) Action.

(C) Bargaining.

(D) Hopelessness.

(23) A sodium-restricted diet is ordered for people with:

(A) Pancreatic disease.

(B) Malaria.

(C) Kidney disease.

(D) Splenic disease.

(24) CNA Tina must help a 70-year-old stroke survivor with elimination. The patient is unstable, and Tina needs to be in the restroom with her. How can the CNA provide the patient with privacy?

(A) She can turn her back on the patient.

(B) She can cover her face.

(C) She can cover the patient's face.

(D) She can leave the patient alone in the room.

(25) A 55-year-old patient develops urinary symptoms. He now urinates more frequently and is not able to hold his urine for long. He also has a low-grade fever. Which of the following investigations will most benefit the patient?

(A) Urine microscopy and culture.

(B) Fasting lipid profile.

(C) Urine protein.

(D) Urine electrolytes.

(26) The pain of appendicitis is usually described as:

(A) Acute.

(B) Chronic.

(C) Subacute.

(D) Acute on chronic.

(27) A 60-year-old patient can't keep food on a spoon due to unsteadiness. Which of the following may help the patient?

(A) Use of his bare hands.

(B) A spork.

(C) A wooden spoon.

(D) A plastic spoon.

(28) Which of the following is not part of grooming?

(A) Nail care.

(B) Hair care.

(C) Tattooing.

(D) Face care.

(29) A 34-year-old man with schizophrenia is brought to the ER after he tried to harm his neighbor. He heard a voice that he now attributes to the neighbor and says it cursed and criticized him. The voice is:

(A) A delusion.

(B) Anxiety.

(C) A hallucination.

(D) Depression.

(30) A 65-year-old woman sometimes forgets things like where she placed her phone. She is healthy and can manage her personal finances fine by herself. Which of the following is true about the woman?

(A) She has dementia.

(B) This is a normal part of aging.

(C) She has delirium.

(D) She has amnesia.

(31) All of the following approaches help to prevent pressure ulcers, except:
(A) Good skin care.
(B) Movement.
(C) Good nutrition and fluid intake.
(D) Long bed rest.

(32) Which of the following beliefs about HIV is false?
(A) It can be contracted from casual contact.
(B) It can be contracted from sexual intercourse.
(C) The risk is higher in homosexuals.
(D) It can be contracted from a blood transfusion.

(33) A 46-year-old patient with asthma is admitted to the respiratory unit. Which of the following actions is best for the CNA to take in the management of this patient?
(A) Help the patient exercise every day.
(B) Help the patient cut down on food.
(C) Help the patient cut down on alcohol.
(D) Help the patient identify triggers.

(34) Which of the following is not a treatment modality for cancer?
(A) Radiotherapy.
(B) Chemotherapy.
(C) Surgery.
(D) Conservative management.

(35) What is an emotional support strategy that can be carried out by family members?
(A) Ignore the patient and give them time to heal.
(B) Avoid social interactions with the patient.
(C) Provide for the patient's basic needs.
(D) Leave the responsibility for the patient's care to the CNA.

(36) What is a key action when caring for a patient with a skin problem?
(A) Apply any over-the-counter ointment without consulting a nurse.
(B) Regularly inspect the skin for changes and report them to the nursing staff.
(C) Advise the patient to use hot water baths to soothe the skin.
(D) Ignore minor skin issues as they are not serious.

(37) Clara is a 22-year-old client who has a history of trauma and abuse. How can a CNA help this client meet her need for love and belonging?
(A) Report the situation to the police.
(B) Report the situation to Clara's family members.
(C) Help the client to learn trust and connect with others in a safe and healthy way.
(D) Do nothing, as Clara will outgrow the problems over time.

(38) How should you handle a patient's dietary restrictions?
(A) Ignore the restrictions as they are not medically important.
(B) Offer the patient whatever food they prefer, regardless of restrictions.
(C) Strictly adhere to the prescribed dietary restrictions and report any concerns.
(D) Encourage the patient to experiment with forbidden foods occasionally.

(39) A 70-year-old woman says she feels less intimate with her husband lately. She says they don't have sex as often as they used to, and they don't cuddle or kiss as much either. What is the most likely reason for this patient's relationship changes?
(A) Normal changes due to aging.
(B) Health problems.
(C) Medications.
(D) Stress.

(40) A common disease that cannot be transmitted in a healthcare facility is:
(A) Tuberculosis.
(B) HIV/AIDS.
(C) Influenza.
(D) Stroke.

(41) Skin tears do not result from:
(A) Blunt force.
(B) Scrapes.
(C) Skin rub.
(D) Surgical incisions.

(42) A 60-year-old man had a below-knee amputation of the right leg. He needs a CNA's help with:

(A) Feeding.

(B) Diet.

(C) Mobility.

(D) Pain management.

(43) What is an appropriate care approach for a nurse aide when assisting a patient with weak ribs?

(A) Encourage the patient to perform high-impact exercises to strengthen the ribs.

(B) Assist with gentle movements and provide support during coughing or deep breathing.

(C) Bind the chest tightly to prevent rib movement.

(D) Ignore the condition as it does not affect patient care.

(44) What are effective measures that can be taken to prevent the spread of diseases in a healthcare facility?

(A) Proper handwashing techniques.

(B) Use of PPE.

(C) Isolation of infected patients.

(D) All of the above.

(45) Some of the major side effects of restraints are:

(A) Death.

(B) Depression.

(C) Bruises.

(D) All of the above.

(46) One way to ensure every patient is adequately monitored is:

(A) Task delegation.

(B) Properly planned schedules.

(C) Security systems.

(D) All of the above.

(47) One advantage of bedrails is that:
(A) They provide safety even at night.
(B) They are not mobile.
(C) They help patients to move around.
(D) They do not really prevent falls.

(48) A patient with tuberculosis does not want to be isolated. What should the CNA tell the patient?
(A) Isolation is not discrimination.
(B) Isolation helps to keep others in the health facility safe.
(C) Isolation is optional.
(D) Both A and B.

(49) What bones form the axial skeleton?
(A) The skull.
(B) The vertebral column.
(C) The bony thorax.
(D) All of the above.

(50) What percentage of the blood is plasma?
(A) 45%.
(B) 50%.
(C) 55%.
(D) 60%.

(51) Which of the following is not important in a patient with breathing difficulties?
(A) Oxygen cylinders.
(B) Nasal prongs.
(C) Urinary catheter.
(D) Pulse oximeter.

(52) What is the normal respiratory cycle in an adult?
(A) 5 to 10 cycles per minute.
(B) 12 to 22 cycles per minute.
(C) 2 to 10 cycles per minute.
(D) 16 to 28 cycles per minute.

(53) Where is chyme formed?
(A) The small intestine.
(B) The stomach.
(C) The large intestine.
(D) The cecum.

(54) What position should a four-year-old child who suffers convulsions be placed in?
(A) Recumbent position.
(B) Left lateral position.
(C) Right lateral position.
(D) Supine position.

(55) A 45-year-old man recently had a lumbar puncture on account of suspected meningitis. How should he be positioned in bed?
(A) With the head of the bed raised about 45 degrees.
(B) With the foot of the bed raised 30 degrees.
(C) With the bed completely flat for at least eight hours after the procedure.
(D) In the Sim's position.

(56) Which of the following is the correct procedure to follow when a patient is bathed?
(A) Wash the eyes from the outer to the inner aspect.
(B) Expose both of the patient's arms at once.
(C) Use a different area of the washcloth for each stroke.
(D) All of the above.

(57) When a bed bath is given, CNAs should:
(A) Avoid contact between the gloves and themselves.
(B) Avoid contact between the used linens and the client's clothing.
(C) Avoid over-extension of the client's joints.
(D) All of the above.

(58) What is the first thing that should be done once urine has been measured?
(A) Return the container to its designated spot.
(B) Return the bedpan to its designated spot.
(C) Empty the contents of the container.
(D) Record the urine output.

(59) What is an important consideration when caring for a patient with a larynx condition?
(A) Encouraging the patient to speak loudly and frequently to strengthen the larynx.
(B) Providing care that minimizes the need for the patient to use their voice.
(C) Teaching the patient to breathe through their mouth constantly.
(D) Advising the patient to consume alcohol to relax the throat muscles.

(60) Which of the following measurements involve weight?
(A) OFC.
(B) MUAC.
(C) BMI.
(D) All of the above.

(61) In which of the following conditions is weight important?
(A) Diabetes.
(B) Obesity.
(C) Arthritis.
(D) All of the above.

(62) In dorsiflexion, what happens to the toes?
(A) They point up.
(B) They point down.
(C) They point sideways.
(D) They point straight.

(63) What is a key care consideration when assisting a patient with a pharynx disorder?
(A) Encourage the patient to consume dry and coarse foods to scrub the pharynx.
(B) Assist the patient with gentle swallowing exercises, if recommended.
(C) Instruct the patient to avoid drinking fluids to reduce pharynx irritation.
(D) Recommend shouting as a method to strengthen the pharynx.

(64) How should the joints be moved during ROM?
(A) Fast.
(B) Slowly.
(C) Gently.
(D) Both B and C.

(65) Where is the resting position of the arm?
(A) By the side of the head.
(B) At ear level.
(C) At the side of the body.
(D) All of the above.

(66) What should you do when assisting a patient with a finger tendon injury?
(A) Encourage the patient to avoid using their hand completely to speed up healing.
(B) Assist with prescribed hand exercises and ensure proper positioning of the hand.
(C) Advise the patient to engage in heavy lifting to strengthen the hand muscles.
(D) Apply heat continuously to the injured finger.

(67) On what side of the bed should the side rail be raised?
(A) On the side opposite where the patient will be turned.
(B) On the side on which the patient will be turned.
(C) At the head of the bed.
(D) At the foot of the bed.

(68) How should a CNA support the head of a patient who is being turned?
(A) Use the side rails.
(B) Use the curtains.
(C) Use folded clothes.
(D) Use a pillow.

(69) What should be placed under the perineal area before it is washed?
(A) Gloves.
(B) A stack of clothes.
(C) A disposable container.
(D) A linen protector.

(70) How much exposure is sufficient when a CNA provides catheter care for a female?

(A) Head and neck.

(B) Head to toe.

(C) Waist to feet.

(D) Hip to knee.

Test 6: Answers and Explanations

(1) (D) Provision of intravenous access.

CNAs have a duty to protect patients' safety, privacy, and personal dignity. However, it is beyond the scope of their profession to perform procedures (intravenous access, cannulation, catheterization, medications) meant for more qualified health personnel, such as nurses, doctors, and phlebotomists.

(2) (B) Occupational Safety and Health Administration.

The Occupational Safety and Health Administration provides regulations and guidelines that guide the protection of workers.

(3) (B) To enhance lung function after surgery or during lung illness.

A spirometer is a device used to measure the volume of air inhaled and exhaled by the lungs. For patients who have undergone surgery, particularly thoracic or abdominal surgery, or those suffering from lung illnesses, using a spirometer can be an important part of their care. It helps in exercising the lungs, preventing complications such as pneumonia, and monitoring their lung function.

(4) (B) Handwashing.

Handwashing is the most important infection prevention and control strategy. It helps to protect against the transfer of contact infections. Although PPE helps to control the spread of infection, handwashing is more important.

(5) (D) Lay the patient in the left lateral position and call 911.

This patient is having convulsions, characterized by jerky movements of the extremities. Convulsions are a result of neurons that misfire in the brain. The initial goal of management when a patient convulses outside of a healthcare setting is to help reduce the risk of complications like aspiration by laying the patient in the left lateral position before calling for help.

(6) (B) Severe central chest pain that radiates to the arms, diaphoresis.

Myocardial infarction is a life-threatening condition caused by obstruction to the coronary blood flow. It causes severe central chest pain that radiates to the arm. There is also associated nausea, vomiting, and a feeling of impending doom. It must be treated as an emergency.

(7) (A) Bedsores.

Bedsores are a complication of prolonged immobilization. They occur mostly in areas with bony prominences. They begin first as non-blanchable erythema on the skin. Later, they progress to open sores. Bedsores can be mostly prevented when patients are turned regularly and/or specialized devices and beds are used.

(8) (D) The patient starts the urine stream, stops, then restarts and collects the sample.

Mid-stream collection is the gold-standard urine collection for microscopy, culture, and sensitivity. To collect midstream urine, the patient is instructed to start the urine stream and then stop. The patient then restarts the urine stream and collects the sample with the clean-catch method. This helps to prevent contaminants.

(9) (C) Greet the patient and ask how she would like to be addressed.

A CNA is expected to greet patients and ask how they would like to be addressed before a professional discussion is started with them. This ensures that the patient's name and pronouns are confirmed. It is wrong to assume gender and name based on physical looks.

(10) (C) Electrocardiogram.

Myocardial infarction is a life-threatening complication of coronary artery disease. Coronary artery disease occurs from thrombosis and occlusion of coronary vessels. This presents with angina pain and, in severe cases, myocardial infarction. An electrocardiogram is used to diagnose myocardial infarction.

(11) (C) Initiation of cardiopulmonary resuscitation.

Initiation of cardiopulmonary resuscitation is life-sustaining care, which is prohibited in an individual with a DNR-CC. Administration of oxygen, pain medications, and supportive care can be done.

(12) (B) Provide for the girl's privacy.

Generally, older and adolescent children are very concerned about privacy. Body image and how they are perceived by others are very important to them. As a result, adolescents can become very distressed by injury or disability, especially if it causes a change in body image.

(13) (A) Tinnitus.

Tinnitus is a persistent ringing in the ear. It may be a symptom of an underlying heart condition. Deafness is a severe loss of hearing. Presbycusis is hearing loss associated with aging.

(14) (C) Swollen legs.

Symptoms of acute asthma exacerbation include a cough that worsens, wheezing, respiratory difficulty, and sometimes, chest pain. Severe cases may present with a silent chest and loss of consciousness. Swollen legs may be from edema and are usually a sign of congestive cardiac failure, chronic kidney disease, etc.

(15) (C) Mobility.

Before a patient is moved or transferred from one point in the health facility to another, it is essential to determine the individual's degree of mobility. Also, the CNA should find out about any specific movement problems. This helps to know the instructions to give patients on how they can help to make the transfer easier.

(16) (C) Positioning aids.

Patients who are frail and sick may require support to stabilize them and prevent falls. Positioning aids are designed to provide that function. Sheets, pneumatic beds, and bed cradles are not used to aid positioning in bed.

(17) (C) Dental caries.

Dental caries are a complication of poor oral care. Patients in assisted living facilities should be helped to achieve optimum oral hygiene to reduce the risk of oral diseases such as cavities and severe oral infections such as dentoalveolar space infections and Ludwig angina. Ludwig angina can cause severe oral complications.

(18) (A) Diet.

Diabetes mellitus is a metabolic disorder that is characterized by hyperglycemia. Hyperglycemia can be treated nonpharmacologically in mild cases. Dietary modifications and regular exercise, in addition to the cessation of alcohol and smoking, can help to control blood sugar.

(19) (D) Pain from a fall.

Acute pain usually occurs suddenly in response to injury or illness (for example, the pain of a broken bone or appendicitis). Chronic pain, however, lasts a long time (beyond six months). It can be constant or intermittent (off and on) and ranges in intensity from mild to severe. Examples of chronic pain include cancer pain, osteoarthritic pain, and osteoporotic pain.

(20) (C) Denial.

Denial is one way patients deal with information that is difficult to accept. It allows the person to put information aside until they are emotionally ready to deal with it. Other emotions that can be expressed by a dying person include hope, acceptance, anger, sadness, and grief.

(21) (A) Encouraged to speak about their needs and feelings.

Family members of a dying person should be encouraged to speak about their needs and feelings. A dying person should not be left alone. Family members should also be encouraged not to give up participation in the care of a dying person.

(22) (D) Hopelessness.

Hopelessness and worthlessness are two features of severe depression. When patients reach the stage of hopelessness, they may contemplate suicide. Patients at this stage should be further evaluated and managed to prevent self-harm.

(23) (C) Kidney disease.

Because of renal impairment, people with kidney disease have difficulty with the excretion of electrolytes. They are also prone to developing hypertension. Thus, sodium-restricted diets are common for such patients.

(24) (A) She can turn her back on the patient.

When patients eliminate, it is important to give them some privacy. However, some patients need the presence of a CNA in the restroom because they are unstable. When possible, CNAs should turn away from patients when they relieve themselves.

(25) (A) Urine microscopy and culture.

This patient with urinary frequency, urgency, and low-grade fever most likely has a UTI. UTIs occur due to the invasion of the urinary tract by microorganisms. Diagnosis is usually by urine culture microscopy of a midstream clean-catch urine sample.

(26) (A) Acute.

Acute appendicitis causes a sudden onset of right lower abdominal pain that is associated with nausea and vomiting. The pain may rapidly progress to severe abdominal pain or resolve on its own without treatment. Acute pain starts and resolves within six months.

(27) (B) A spork.

A spork is a specialized form of spoon with sharp edges. It combines the unique characteristics of a spoon and fork and can help patients who cannot maintain the required steadiness to eat with a normal spoon. A swivel fork or spoon is another utensil that is similar in function to a spork.

(28) (C) Tattooing.

Tattooing is not a component of grooming. It is associated with medical risks such as the transmission of bloodborne viral and bacterial infections.

(29) (C) A hallucination.

Hallucinations are experiences that a patient has in response to an unreal stimulus. Delusions are unusual beliefs that are unfounded and impractical. Both delusions and hallucinations are features of psychotic disorders such as schizophrenia and mania.

(30) (B) This is a normal part of aging.

Normal aging is associated with increased forgetfulness and other subtle changes in memory. This patient can manage her finances on her own, which shows that she does not have a significant intellectual impairment. The other options listed are pathological.

(31) (D) Long bed rest.

Those at risk of pressure ulcers include immobilized patients, patients with fractures, neurological injuries, the elderly, etc. Such patients should be turned regularly in bed, have regular skin care, and be encouraged to move out of bed if possible.

(32) (A) It can be contracted from casual contact.

This is incorrect. HIV cannot be contracted from casual contact. It can also be contracted from sexual intercourse, blood transfusion, sharing of sharps, and use of unsterilized sharp equipment. The risk is higher in homosexuals.

(33) (D) Help the patient identify triggers.

In the management of acute asthma exacerbations, medical personnel need to collaborate with the patient to identify triggers.

(34) (D) Conservative management.

Cancer is the second most common cause of death globally. It is a deadly disease that should be treated as early as possible when diagnosed. It is not treated by a conservative approach. Cancer is treated by chemotherapy, radiotherapy, and surgery.

(35) (C) Provide for the patient's basic needs.

Family members are encouraged to visit patients, support them, and provide for their basic needs as well.

(36) (B) Regularly inspect the skin for changes and report them to the nursing staff.

Regularly inspect the skin for any changes or signs of worsening conditions and report these observations to the nursing staff. This allows for timely intervention and management of the skin condition.

(37) (C) Help the client to learn trust and connect with others in a safe and healthy way.

A CNA can help Clara meet her need for love and belonging by assisting her with learning to trust and connect with others in a safe and healthy manner. Building a sense of trust and establishing positive relationships are important steps for someone who is trying to recover from trauma and abuse.

(38) (C) Strictly adhere to the prescribed dietary restrictions and report any concerns.

Dietary restrictions are often prescribed for medical reasons, such as allergies, specific health conditions, or recovery from surgery. It is essential to strictly follow these guidelines to ensure the patient's safety and well-being.

(39) (B) Health problems.

As people age, they are likely to have health problems. Health problems can have a significant impact on intimacy. For example, conditions such as arthritis, heart disease, and diabetes can make sex difficult or painful.

(40) (D) Stroke.

Stroke is not a communicable disease. It is due to a blockage of one of the arteries in the brain. Tuberculosis can be transmitted via droplets. HIV/AIDS can be transmitted by sharps, and influenza can also be transmitted by air droplets and personal contact.

(41) (D) Surgical incision.

Skin tears occur when there is a break in the skin. The skin layer can be partially removed or totally lifted. Skin tears can result from trauma or blunt force, a cut or scrape (known as shearing), or friction that results from skin that rubs.

(42) (C) Mobility.

A patient with a below-knee amputation of the right leg will need help with mobility until he learns a new way to maneuver.

(43) (B) Assist with gentle movements and provide support during coughing or deep breathing.

It is important for a nurse aide to assist with gentle movements to avoid causing pain or further injury. Supporting the patient during coughing or deep breathing can help minimize discomfort and facilitate these necessary actions.

(44) (D) All of the above.

All the measures listed are important to prevent the spread of diseases in the health facility.

(45) (D) All of the above.

Restraints can have complications. Death can result from drug overdoses or side effects of some of the drugs used to sedate patients. Bruises can result from physical restraints if the patient struggles, and depression can also be an emotional consequence in a patient who is restrained.

(46) (D) All of the above.

Task delegation ensures that work is spread evenly among healthcare staff. Properly planned schedules make sure that everyone is catered to, and security systems help provide an extra layer of monitoring.

(47) (A) They provide safety, even at night.

Once bedrails are set up, they can prevent falls at night, when patients may turn or toss in their sleep or if they attempt to stand while unassisted.

(48) (D) Both A and B.

Isolation is not discrimination against the patient. It is just a measure to keep healthcare workers and other patients safe.

(49) (D) All of the above.

The axial skeleton forms the longitudinal axis of the body. It comprises the skull, the vertebral column, and the bony thorax. Eighty bones altogether form the axial skeleton in humans.

(50) (C) 55%.

Fifty-five percent of the blood is formed by plasma. Forty-five percent of the blood comprises elements like the white blood cells, red blood cells, and thrombocytes.

(51) (C) Urinary catheter.

This is incorrect. A patient with breathing difficulties will need nasal prongs, oxygen, and a pulse oximeter to measure the level of oxygen in the blood.

(52) (B) 12 to 22 cycles per minute.

The normal respiratory cycle is 12 to 22 cycles per minute (cpm). Cycles higher than this range in normal respiration are termed tachypnea. Cycles less than this are referred to as bradypnea.

(53) (B) The stomach.

Chyme is formed in the stomach from the mixture of digested food and stomach chemicals.

(54) (B) Left lateral position.

A convulsing child should be placed in the left lateral position. This helps to prevent the aspiration of secretions.

(55) (C) With the bed completely flat for at least eight hours after the procedure.

To reduce the risk of a headache after a lumbar puncture, the patient should lie flat in bed for a minimum of eight hours after the procedure.

(56) (C) Use a different area of the washcloth for each stroke.

The correct procedure to follow when bathing a patient includes using a different area of the washcloth for each stroke. This practice is important to prevent the spread of bacteria. By using a clean section of the washcloth for each stroke, the risk of recontaminating areas that have already been cleaned is minimized.

(57) (D) All of the above.

There should be no contact between the gloves and the CNA and no contact between the patient's clothes and any soiled clothes. The CNA should also move all joints naturally and gently while the patient is bathed.

(58) (D) Record the urine output.

Once urine has been measured, the first thing that should be done is to record the urine output. Accurate recording of urine output is important when monitoring a patient's fluid balance and kidney function.

(59) (B) Providing care that minimizes the need for the patient to use their voice.

For patients with a condition affecting the larynx, such as laryngitis or other voice disorders, it's important to minimize strain on the voice box. This involves providing care that reduces the need for the patient to speak, which can help in the healing process and prevent further irritation.

(60) (C) BMI.

Among the options provided, BMI (Body Mass Index) involves weight. BMI is a measure that uses both weight and height to calculate a numerical value that helps assess whether a person is underweight, normal weight, overweight, or obese. It's calculated by dividing a person's weight in kilograms by their height in meters squared. OFC (Occipital Frontal Circumference) measures the circumference of the head, and is used for infants and young children to assess brain and skull growth. MUAC (Mid-Upper Arm Circumference) measures the circumference of the upper arm and is used to assess nutritional status. These measurements involve dimensions instead of weight.

(61) (D) All of the above.

Weight is important in diabetes, as being obese is a major risk factor. Arthritis is also influenced by weight, and one of the commonly prescribed lifestyle adjustments for arthritis is weight loss.

(62) (A) They point up.

In dorsiflexion, the toes point upwards. Dorsiflexion is the action of moving the foot so that the toes are brought closer to the shin. This movement decreases the angle between the dorsum (top) of the foot and the leg, which results in the toes pointing up towards the shin.

(63) (B) Assist the patient with gentle swallowing exercises, if recommended.

For patients with a pharynx disorder, which can impact swallowing, it's important to assist with any gentle swallowing exercises that have been recommended by a healthcare professional. These exercises can help strengthen the muscles used in swallowing and improve the patient's ability to eat and drink safely.

(64) (D) Both B and C.

During Range of Motion (ROM) exercises, the joints should be moved both slowly and gently. Moving the joints slowly ensures that the full range of motion is utilized without causing strain or injury. It allows for better control of the movement and minimizes the risk of causing pain or discomfort to the patient.

(65) (C) At the side of the body.

The resting position of the arm is at the side of the body. This is the natural position the arm returns to when it is not actively performing a movement.

(66) (B) Assist with prescribed hand exercises and ensure proper positioning of the hand.

For a patient with a finger tendon injury, it is important to assist with any hand exercises that have been prescribed. These exercises are important for maintaining the flexibility and strength of the hand.

(67) (A) On the side opposite where the patient will be turned.

The side rail should be raised on the side opposite where the patient will be turned. This provides safety for the patient and ensures they do not roll or fall out of the bed during the turning process.

(68) (D) Use a pillow.

When a patient is turned, the CNA should place a pillow under the head of the patient to act as a support.

(69) (D) A linen protector.

The linen protector serves to protect the patient's sheets from getting wet, contaminated, or dirty.

(70) (D) Hip to knee.

It is key to only expose the patient as much as is needed. To perform catheter care, only the areas that surround the catheter need exposure, between the hip and knees.

Test 7: Questions

(1) What is the minimum number of hours required to train as a certified CNA per federal regulations?

(A) 60.

(B) 120.

(C) 150.

(D) 75.

(2) What is not one of the principles of medical ethics?

(A) Justice.

(B) Nonmaleficence.

(C) Autonomy.

(D) Simplicity.

(3) A CNA wants to check trends in a patient's vital signs. Which of the following forms will be most helpful?

(A) Nursing notes.

(B) Care plan.

(C) Flow sheet.

(D) Case notes.

(4) Standard precautions should be used:

(A) Only when high-risk patients are attended to.

(B) At all times.

(C) Only when in the operating room.

(D) Only when young patients are attended to.

(5) A CNA's colleague suffers a cut to the hand. The laceration bleeds profusely. What should be done to help the person?

(A) Wear gloves.

(B) Wash both the person's hands.

(C) Wash the wound.

(D) Apply a dressing to the wound.

(6) Which of the following sets of vital signs is out of range for a normal adult?
(A) Blood pressure of 110/80 mmHg.
(B) Temperature of 99 F.
(C) Respiration of 16 cycles/min.
(D) Pulse of 110 beats/min.

(7) What is the first sign of a pressure ulcer?
(A) Scaly skin.
(B) Red skin.
(C) Dark pigmentation.
(D) Open wound.

(8) Mr. Tom is a 67-year-old man admitted to the ward after a surgical procedure. He has a urethral catheter. He develops fever, dysuria, and urinary frequency on postoperative day 10 and is diagnosed with a UTI. Which of the following most likely increased his risk of infection?
(A) Age.
(B) Sex.
(C) Surgery.
(D) Indwelling catheter.

(9) Admission refers to:
(A) Entry to a ward.
(B) A person's formal entry into a healthcare setting.
(C) A person's exit from a healthcare setting.
(D) Both B and C.

(10) What is a classical angina symptom?
(A) Epigastric pain.
(B) Right hypochondriac pain.
(C) Central chest pain unrelieved by nitroglycerin.
(D) Central chest pain relieved by nitroglycerin.

(11) Cardiopulmonary resuscitation is an example of:
(A) Palliative care.
(B) Supportive care.
(C) Life-sustaining care.
(D) Hospice care.

(12) The vital signs of a child are as follows:
Pulse rate: 140 beats/min
Respiratory rate: 50 cycles/min.
These findings are most consistent with a child of what age?
(A) 0–3 months.
(B) 3–6 months.
(C) 6–12 months.
(D) 1–3 years.

(13) Which medical condition causes tingling sensations in the feet?
(A) Hypertension.
(B) Asthma.
(C) Diabetes.
(D) Heart failure.

(14) A patient with chronic bronchitis requires help with:
(A) Respiratory secretions.
(B) Bowel movements.
(C) Urination.
(D) Perineal care.

(15) What is an important piece of equipment used to prevent the worsening of a neck injury when a patient is moved?
(A) Neck collar.
(B) Minerva.
(C) Neck bandage.
(D) Neck ultrasound scan.

(16) A CNA must help a 76-year-old patient with mouth care. She rinses the patient's mouth with a liquid substance before and after the mouth care. What is the substance?
(A) Saltwater.
(B) Chlorinated water.
(C) Toothpaste.
(D) Diluted mouthwash.

(17) What is a possible complication of poor transfer methods?
(A) Infection.
(B) Falls.
(C) Anxiety.
(D) Depression.

(18) Which dietary measures can help control hypertension?
(A) Increased salt consumption.
(B) Increased fat consumption.
(C) Increased sugar consumption.
(D) Increased fruit and vegetable consumption.

(19) Mrs. Nancy complains of pain to the CNA. The CNA reports the pain to the nurse. A fact not included in this report is:
(A) The location of the pain.
(B) The frequency of the pain.
(C) The drugs the CNA would like to use to treat the pain.
(D) The intensity of the pain.

(20) All of the following are signs an individual is approaching death except:
(A) Rapid, weak, and irregular pulse.
(B) Decreased blood pressure.
(C) Cool, moist, and pale skin.
(D) Warm, dry, and pink skin.

(21) A 50-year-old woman experiences moments when she is excessively elated and other moments when she is excessively sad and teary. The woman most likely has:

(A) Depression.

(B) Mania.

(C) Bipolar disorder.

(D) Grief.

(22) What is a symptom of attention-deficit hyperactivity disorder?

(A) Low mood.

(B) Inattention.

(C) Anger.

(D) Anxiety.

(23) A 60-year-old patient is served lunch. What is the best approach for the CNA to take?

(A) Ask about the amount of help the patient needs.

(B) Feed the patient.

(C) Drop the food off and attend to other things.

(D) Tell the patient to eat as fast as possible.

(24) A 60-year-old patient is able to get out of bed but unable to move to the toilet for defecation. Which device will be most helpful to the patient?

(A) Portable commode.

(B) Urinal.

(C) Bedpan.

(D) Catheter.

(25) Which of the following is wrong about catheter care?

(A) The bag should be placed on the floor.

(B) The drainage bag should be secured to a bedframe.

(C) The tubing should be secured to the patient's thigh.

(D) The collection bag should be regularly drained.

(26) Which of the following is an indication for stool specimen collection?
(A) New-onset diarrhea.
(B) Constipation.
(C) Cough.
(D) New-onset fever.

(27) A 60-year-old stroke survivor can't hold a spoon steady. Which of the following may benefit the patient?
(A) Utensil holder.
(B) Plastic spoon.
(C) Food tray.
(D) Spork.

(28) Which of the following is not true about grooming?
(A) It improves a sense of self-worth.
(B) It prevents infections and infestations.
(C) It improves the patient's sense of belonging.
(D) It improves the patient's appetite.

(29) A 45-year-old woman does not drink water produced in a nearby factory because she believes all the water has been poisoned. So, she travels a few miles to buy "clean" water. This is best described as:
(A) Suspicion.
(B) Delusion.
(C) Hallucination.
(D) Depression.

(30) Mr. Caleb is a 44-year-old man who can bear weight but needs support on both sides. He is a survivor of a car accident. What would be the best mobility device for him to use?
(A) A walker.
(B) A cane.
(C) Crutches.
(D) A wheelchair.

(31) Patients with osteoarthritis usually experience:
(A) Acute pain.
(B) Chronic pain.
(C) Pulselessness.
(D) Paresthesia.

(32) A 54-year-old trauma patient uses a device installed over his bed to facilitate easy movement and repositioning. This device is called a:
(A) Trapeze.
(B) Transfer belt.
(C) Movement aid.
(D) Brace.

(33) Which of the following is a symptom of Parkinson's disease?
(A) Weight gain.
(B) Tremors.
(C) Blindness.
(D) Weight loss.

(34) An extremely depressed patient may contemplate:
(A) Anger.
(B) Suicide.
(C) Hope.
(D) Denial.

(35) What does systolic pressure represent in a blood pressure reading?
(A) The pressure in the arteries when the heart relaxes between beats.
(B) The pressure in the arteries when the heart is actively pumping blood.
(C) The number of heartbeats per minute.
(D) The level of cholesterol in the blood.

(36) Mrs. Paulina, a 65-year-old woman, is a patient in a nursing home. She raises concerns about loneliness. What can a CNA do to enhance this patient's emotional and mental wellness?

(A) Do not discuss the patient's feelings with her.

(B) Encourage interactions, play games, do role play, or set up movie nights.

(C) Give her medications to sleep more.

(D) Discharge her from the health facility.

(37) A 16-year-old male patient is struggling with low self-esteem and feelings of inadequacy. How can a therapist help this client?

(A) Take the client out and force him to interact.

(B) Ignore the problem as it will resolve with age.

(C) Identify and challenge the client's negative self-beliefs and help him develop a more positive and realistic image of himself.

(D) Report the situation to the client's parents.

(38) What is the term for the feeling of loneliness and isolation that can occur with aging?

(A) Empty nest syndrome.

(B) Anomie.

(C) Bereavement.

(D) Anxiety.

(39) When is it most appropriate to use a transfer belt?

(A) When the patient is resting in bed to keep them secure.

(B) During patient transfers and ambulation to provide support and safety.

(C) Only when the patient requests it as a comfort measure.

(D) To restrain a patient who is being uncooperative.

(40) Which healthcare practice effectively prevents or limits the transmission of tuberculosis in the healthcare environment?

(A) Patient isolation.

(B) Handwashing.

(C) Disinfection.

(D) Vaccination.

(41)A CNA observes that the patient she is managing has a wound dressing that smells bad. What is the next course of action?

(A) Open the dressing to check it.

(B) Inform the nurse.

(C) Commence antibiotics.

(D) All of the above.

(42) One way to prevent a UTI in a 50-year-old male patient with a urinary catheter is to:

(A) Insert the catheter septically.

(B) Change the catheter when needed.

(C) Administer broad-spectrum antibiotics.

(D) All of the above.

(43) What is the best response to a patient who has been vomiting for the past three hours?

(A) Administer first aid.

(B) Encourage the patient to drink more fluids.

(C) Report to the charge nurse.

(D) All of the above.

(44) A patient is aggressive and uses foul language on other patients. What should a CNA first do?

(A) Attempt to pacify the patient.

(B) Administer sedatives.

(C) Call the charge nurse.

(D) Restrain the patient.

(45) One major guideline in the use of restraints is:

(A) They must be absolutely necessary.

(B) They must only be used as a last resort.

(C) They must be removed regularly.

(D) All of the above.

(46) When is it most appropriate to position a patient's bed in a high position?
(A) When the patient is sleeping.
(B) To facilitate patient care such as changing linens or performing procedures.
(C) After the patient has eaten a meal.
(D) As a default position for all patients for easier visibility.

(47) A CNA who cares about patient comfort must pay close attention to:
(A) Patient positioning.
(B) Hygienic practices.
(C) Diet.
(D) All of the above.

(48) A 50-year-old woman who suffers from sepsis exhibits antibiotic resistance. What is a major risk factor for antibiotic resistance?
(A) Serious infection.
(B) Indiscriminate antibiotic use.
(C) Pain.
(D) Severe injury.

(49) What type of muscle is found in the intestine?
(A) Voluntary muscle.
(B) Smooth muscle.
(C) Cardiac muscle.
(D) All of the above.

(50) What is the most important function of the red blood cells?
(A) They give blood color.
(B) They increase blood count.
(C) They transport oxygen.
(D) All of the above.

(51) Which bronchus is longer?
(A) The right bronchus.
(B) The left bronchus.
(C) Both are the same length.
(D) All of the above.

(52) A patient with heart failure who experiences breathing difficulties will benefit from placement in the:

(A) Sim's position.

(B) Recumbent position.

(C) Trendelenburg position.

(D) Orthopneic position.

(53) Chyle is formed in the:

(A) Small intestine.

(B) Stomach.

(C) Large intestine.

(D) Cecum.

(54) Which of these drugs should be made available on an emergency tray to abort seizures?

(A) Paraldehyde.

(B) Diazepam.

(C) Adrenaline.

(D) Both A and B.

(55) In the management of a 60-year-old patient with dementia, what is key about the care plan?

(A) The patient should have a different schedule every day.

(B) The patient should have consistent times for activities.

(C) The patient should have a lot of activities.

(D) All of the above.

(56) When a catheter is cleaned, a CNA should not:

(A) Apply soap to a wet washcloth.

(B) Ensure the signaling device is close.

(C) Tug at the catheter.

(D) Hold the catheter at the meatus.

(57) How much of the catheter nearest to the meatus should be cleaned?
(A) At least two inches.
(B) At least four inches.
(C) At least six inches.
(D) At least eight inches.

(58) In what direction should the catheter be cleaned?
(A) Toward the meatus.
(B) Away from the meatus.
(C) Forward and backward.
(D) From side to side.

(59) What are the steps to clean a catheter?
(A) Use a new part of the washcloth for each different stroke.
(B) Empty, rinse, and dry the basins used.
(C) Dispose of soiled linen appropriately.
(D) All of the above.

(60) Which step is incorrect when foot care is provided?
(A) Check the water temperature.
(B) Put on clean gloves.
(C) Apply soap to the patient's feet.
(D) Place the basin in a comfortable position.

(61) How can a CNA wash in between the toes when foot care is provided to a patient?
(A) Lift the patient's foot from the water to wash in between the toes.
(B) Wash the foot inside the basin of water.
(C) Wash the foot after drying it.
(D) Do not ever wash a patient's feet.

(62) Which of the following statements is false when a CNA provides foot care?
(A) The client's bare foot should be placed in the water.
(B) The procedure should be explained first to the client.
(C) The foot should be thoroughly rinsed, including between the toes.
(D) Lotion should be applied to the top and bottom of the foot, including between the toes.

(63) Where should the towel be placed during mouth care?
(A) In the patient's mouth.
(B) On the patient's head.
(C) Below the patient's jaw.
(D) Across the patient's chest.

(64) Where should the emesis basin be placed?
(A) Close to the patient's neck.
(B) Close to the patient's chest.
(C) Close to the patient's chin.
(D) By the side of the patient's head.

(65) What parts are cleaned when mouth care is provided?
(A) The tongue.
(B) The teeth.
(C) The gums.
(D) All of the above.

(66) In the provision of perineal care for a female patient, in what direction should the genital area be cleaned?
(A) From back to front.
(B) From front to back.
(C) From side to side.
(D) In a circular pattern.

(67) How should the genital area in females be dried after it is cleaned?
(A) From back to front.
(B) From front to back.
(C) From side to side.
(D) In a centripetal pattern.

(68) How should the rectal area in females be dried after it is cleaned?
(A) From back to front.
(B) From front to back.
(C) From side to side.
(D) In a centripetal pattern.

(69) What should be done before a patient is assisted to stand?

(A) Remove the footrests.

(B) Replace the footrests.

(C) Open the wheels of the wheelchair.

(D) All of the above.

(70) What position should the feet of a patient be in right before they are assisted to stand?

(A) In a curved position.

(B) In a bent position.

(C) Flat on the floor.

(D) In a raised position.

Test 7: Answers and Explanations

(1) (D) 75.

According to federal regulations, a CNA should be trained for a minimum of 75 hours in order to qualify for the certificate exam. However, this is just the minimum acceptable standard. Most institutions and professional bodies train people for much longer.

(2) (D) Simplicity.

The principles of medical ethics refer to a group of guidelines that guide healthcare worker and patient relationships. They help to foster a therapeutic alliance and protect patients from harm. They include justice, autonomy, nonmaleficence, and beneficence.

(3) (C) Flow sheet.

A flow sheet is one of the forms in a patient's medical records. It is where trends in the patient's vital signs and other regularly checked data are recorded for easy access and decision-making. The care plan is where detailed information about patient management and frequency of interventions are recorded.

(4) (B) At all times.

CNAs must ensure they follow standard precaution protocols at all times when in healthcare facilities. This helps to reduce the risk of infection spread, occupational hazards, and other work-related adverse events.

(5) (A) Wear gloves.

When a patient is bleeding, the best initial step is to don gloves to reduce the risk of infection spread. After gloves are donned, a dressing can be applied with pressure directly over the laceration. The pressure helps to stop the bleeding.

(6) (D) Pulse of 110 beats/min.

A patient with a pulse rate of 110 beats/min has a fast pulse. The technical word for fast pulse is tachycardia. A normal pulse is between 60 and 100 beats per minute. Some patients may have a low or high pulse without any disease condition. This is called physiological bradycardia or tachycardia.

(7) (B) Red skin.

Red skin (erythematosus skin) is the first symptom seen in pressure ulcers. Pressure ulcers are common in immobilized patients who spend a long time in bed.

(8) (D) Indwelling catheter.

A catheter-associated urinary tract infection (CAUTI) is a common complication of long-term use of an indwelling catheter. It should be suspected in a patient with an indwelling catheter who develops a fever. Treatment is prompt removal of the indwelling catheter and the administration of antibiotics.

(9) (B) A person's formal entry into a healthcare setting.

Admission refers to the process of a patient's formal entry into a healthcare setting. The setting could be a hospital or a nursing home. During the process of admission, patient details and a baseline physical examination and vital signs are measured and recorded.

(10) (D) Central chest pain relieved by nitroglycerin.

Angina pectoris is one of the complications of coronary artery disease. It presents with recurrent episodes of central chest pain that is relieved by the use of nitroglycerin. Myocardial infarction is more persistent and unrelieved by nitroglycerin.

(11) (C) Life-sustaining care.

Cardiopulmonary resuscitation is life-sustaining care.

(12) (A) 0–3 months.

The vital signs provided are consistent with that of a child of 0–3 months. The normal heart rate of a child of this age is 100–150 beats/min and a normal respiratory rate of 35–55 cycles/min. These figures are higher than the adult values. The normal pulse of an adult is 60–100 beats/min, while the respiratory rate is 16–20 cycles/min.

(13) (C) Diabetes.

Diabetes mellitus is a medical condition characterized by relative or absolute insulin deficiency, which results in hyperglycemia. The symptoms are polyuria, polydipsia, and weight loss. Chronic hyperglycemia damages the sensory system, which causes a tingling sensation (paresthesia).

(14) (A) Respiratory secretions.

Chronic bronchitis is one of the chronic obstructive pulmonary diseases. It is characterized by a persistent cough productive of sputum for at least three months in a year for two consecutive years. Elderly patients with chronic bronchitis require respiratory assistance to clear secretions and prevent aspiration.

(15) (A) Neck collar.

Patients who sustain cervical spine injuries should be given a neck collar to stabilize the spine and prevent further injury during transfer. Oftentimes, a partial cervical injury becomes complete if patients are transferred without neck collars.

(16) (D) Diluted mouthwash.

Mouth care is important in patients who reside in assisted living facilities. This is because poor oral hygiene is associated with several complications in the elderly, such as infective endocarditis, severe mouth infections, etc. During mouth care, the mouth should be washed with diluted mouthwash before and after the procedure.

(17) (B) Falls.

Improper patient instructions and techniques may lead to falls while attempting to move patients. Thus, patients should be properly informed of the reason for the transfer and counseled on how they can help make it easier.

(18) (D) Increased fruit and vegetable consumption.

DASH recommends fruits and vegetables as one of the treatment modalities for hypertension. It includes increased fruits and vegetables in the diet. It has been proven that this approach helps to lower blood pressure significantly.

(19) (C) The drugs the CNA would like to use to treat the pain.

Important facts to report include the location of the pain, the frequency, the intensity, and its character. It is not the client's or CAN's responsibility to determine the care plan or the drugs to be administered.

(20) (D) Warm, dry, and pink skin.

Signs an individual is approaching death may include rapid, weak, or irregular pulse, decreased blood pressure, cool, moist, and pale skin, cool and mottled (patchy discoloration) hands and feet, and incontinence.

(21) (C) Bipolar disorder.

Bipolar affective disorder is characterized by episodes of mania and depression. Mania is associated with excessive elation, confidence, and delusions of grandiosity. Depression is associated with excessive sadness and hopelessness.

(22) (B) Inattention.

Inattention is one of the main symptoms of attention-deficit hyperactivity disorder. The disorder begins in childhood and may persist until adulthood. Patients are easily distracted and inattentive. The symptoms must occur in two different settings (e.g., at school and at home) to make the diagnosis.

(23) (A) Ask about the amount of help the patient needs.

Patients in assisted living facilities often require assistance with nutrition and other aspects of life. Before a CNA provides any help, the best thing to do is confirm the amount of help a patient needs. Some patients can eat on their own if they are provided with the right cutlery.

(24) (A) Portable commode.

A portable commode is a device that helps in elimination for patients who have limited mobility. A patient who can move out of bed but is not strong enough to move independently to the toilet will benefit from a portable commode. Patients who are strong enough should go to the toilet alone or in the company of a CNA.

(25) (A) The bag should be placed on the floor.

With a patient with an indwelling urinary catheter, special care should be taken to ensure that the patient does not develop a UTI. One of the approaches is to secure the catheter tubing in place and ensure that the bag is attached to the bedframe. The bag should never be placed on the floor.

(26) (A) New-onset diarrhea.

New-onset diarrhea can result from chronic inflammatory bowel disease or acute gastroenteritis. Acute gastroenteritis occurs due to an infection of the gastrointestinal tract from parasitic, bacteria, or viral causes. A stool sample collection for microscopy and culture is often required for diagnosis.

(27) (A) Utensil holder.

Patients with different degrees of hand impairments can use a utensil holder to hold spoons, forks, sporks, etc.

(28) (D) It improves the patient's appetite.

Grooming improves a patient's sense of personal hygiene. It also improves the patient's sense of self-esteem and prevents infestation from parasites. It, however, has nothing to do with appetite.

(29) (B) Delusion.

This patient travels several miles to buy water because she believes all the water has been poisoned. The patient is delusional.

(30) (A) A walker.

A walker is specifically made for patients who do not have problems bearing weight but need support on both sides.

(31) (B) Chronic pain.

Osteoarthritis causes chronic pain. It is a non-inflammatory disorder of the joints that is more common in elderly and obese patients. Osteoarthritis is also common following trauma to joints. It presents with chronic joint pain that is usually managed with analgesics.

(32) (A) Trapeze.

A trapeze is a piece of mobility equipment that is installed on the bedframe. It helps to facilitate movement for a patient who is immobilized. Such patients can turn in bed, move their limbs, adjust their sleeping position, or do other things in bed on their own.

(33) (B) Tremors.

Parkinson's disease is a neurological disorder that occurs as a result of the loss of dopaminergic neurons in the basal ganglia of the brain. It presents with movement problems, such as tremors, bradykinesia, shuffling gait, and tremors at rest. Autonomic symptoms may also be seen.

(34) (B) Suicide.

An extremely depressed patient may contemplate suicide because of feelings of worthlessness and hopelessness. Patients with depression should be evaluated for signs of suicidal ideation.

(35) (B) The pressure in the arteries when the heart is actively pumping blood.

Systolic pressure is the top number in a blood pressure reading and represents the amount of pressure in the arteries when the heart muscle contracts and pumps blood out into the arteries. It is a critical indicator of cardiovascular health, as high systolic pressure can indicate an increased risk for heart conditions and other health issues.

(36) (B) Encourage interactions, play games, do role play, or set up movie nights.

Patients in nursing homes or care facilities require emotional support essential for mental health and wellness. This is facilitated through the establishment of quality relationships between caregivers and other patients through meaningful activities. The CNA should encourage role play, games, movie nights, and other forms of social interaction to reduce loneliness and lessen societal withdrawal.

(37) (C) Identify and challenge the client's negative self-beliefs and help him develop a more positive and realistic image of himself.

The CNA can help the client identify and challenge his negative self-beliefs. The CNA can also help the client develop a more positive and realistic self-image.

(38) (B) Anomie.

Anomie is a feeling of social isolation and alienation that can occur in aging. It is often caused by loss of social roles and relationships.

(39) (B) During patient transfers and ambulation to provide support and safety.

A transfer belt is also known as a gait belt. It is used to assist patients who need help with mobility, such as during transfers from a bed to a chair, or while walking. The belt provides a secure way to support the patient and helps prevent falls or injuries during these movements.

(40) (A) Patient isolation.

The spread of tuberculosis can be prevented if a patient is isolated. Then, handwashing and disinfection procedures can be put in place.

(41) (B) Inform the nurse.

The role of the CNA does not extend to the administration of antibiotics or dressing of wounds. So when a patient has a wound that smells bad, the nurse should be informed.

(42) (B) Change the catheter when needed.

One effective way to prevent a urinary tract infection (UTI) for a 50-year-old male patient with a urinary catheter is to change the catheter when needed. Regular and appropriate changing of the catheter is important when minimizing the risk of infection. Catheters can be a source of infection, especially if they are left in place for too long, as bacteria can grow and travel up the catheter into the urinary tract.

(43) (C) Report to the charge nurse.

The best response to a patient who has been vomiting for the past three hours is to report the situation to the charge nurse. Vomiting for an extended period can be a symptom of a more serious underlying condition and should be assessed by a medical professional.

(44) (C) Call the charge nurse.

When dealing with a patient who is aggressive and uses foul language towards others, the first action you should take is to call the charge nurse. The charge nurse can assess the situation and determine the appropriate intervention. This step is important because the behavior might be due to an underlying medical or psychological issue that requires professional evaluation and management.

(45) (D) All of the above.

Restraints must be used only when necessary. They must be used as a last resort and should be removed regularly.

(46) (B) To facilitate patient care such as changing linens or performing procedures.

Raising the bed to a high position is done to bring the patient up to a level that is easier for the caregiver to access, which can be particularly helpful during certain care activities like changing linens, dressing wounds, or performing other procedures. This position helps prevent strain on the caregiver's back and allows for more effective patient care.

(47) (D) All of the above.

CNAs are expected to understand that comfort is a phase of every procedure as it is an aspect of the total care of patients. Comfort is associated with rest, exercise, and the adjustment of the patient's body to the bed and the environment, including patient positioning, hygienic practices, and diet.

(48) (B) Indiscriminate antibiotic use.

Indiscriminate antibiotic risk is a major risk factor for antibiotic resistance.

(49) (B) Smooth muscle.

Smooth muscle is also known as involuntary muscle. It is found in the intestines and other hollow visceral organs in the body, such as the liver and the pancreas. Voluntary muscle is also known as skeletal muscle, while cardiac muscle is found in the heart.

(50) (C) They transport oxygen.

Red blood cells transport oxygen through the hemoglobin. Hemoglobin has a high affinity for oxygen and binds to it, which allows it to be transported to vital tissues in the body.

(51) (B) Left bronchus.

The left bronchus is longer than the right bronchus. It also enters the lung at a greater angle than the lungs. However, the right bronchus is wider than the left bronchus. This increases the risk of aspiration.

(52) (D) Orthopneic position.

In this position, the patient sits upright and leans forward, with pillows in front. This position allows for maximum lung expansion and is useful for patients with difficulty breathing.

(53) (A) Small intestine.

Chyle is formed in the small intestine. It is what is left after excess water and nutrients have been removed from the food as it passes through the gastrointestinal tract.

(54) (B) Diazepam.

Diazepam is the drug that should be made available on an emergency tray for the purpose of aborting seizures. Diazepam is a benzodiazepine that acts as a sedative and anticonvulsant, which makes it effective for stopping active seizure activity. It is commonly used in emergency settings to control or stop seizures due to its rapid onset of action.

(55) (B) The patient should have consistent times for activities.

Routines help dementia patients and every person involved in their care to know what to expect. It adds a form of structure to their lives.

(56) (C) Tug at the catheter.

The catheter is usually held by a balloon inside the bladder when passed through the urethra. Tugging can result in a forceful removal and injury to the bladder and the urethra.

(57) (B) At least four inches.

At least four inches of the catheter should be cleaned. This helps to reduce the risk of contamination and infection since some parts of the catheter will be in contact with the vagina.

(58) (B) Away from the meatus.

When cleaning a catheter, it should be cleaned in a direction that is away from the meatus (the urinary opening). This practice helps to prevent bacteria from coming into the urinary tract, which can cause infections.

(59) (D) All of the above.

A different area should be used for each stroke. The basins should be emptied, rinsed, and dried, and soiled linens should be disposed of appropriately.

(60) (C) Apply soap to the patient's feet.

This is incorrect. Soap should not be applied to the feet. Instead, it should be applied to the wet washcloth that is then used to clean the feet.

(61) (A) Lift the patient's foot from the water to wash in between the toes.

To wash in between the patient's toes, each foot should be lifted out of the water and cleaned, including between the toes.

(62) (D) Lotion should be applied to the top and bottom of the foot, including between the toes.

This is false. Lotion should not be applied between toes because that area can easily be infected with bacteria, fungus, or yeast when there is moisture. So the area between the toes should always be kept dry.

(63) (D) Across the patient's chest.

The cloth towel should be placed across the chest to prevent soiling of the patient's clothes and to soak up any water or secretions from the mouth.

(64) (C) Close to the patient's chin.

The emesis basin should be placed close to the patient's chin when they need to vomit. Positioning the basin near the chin ensures that it is readily accessible and in the most effective position to catch vomit. This placement minimizes the risk of spillage and helps maintain hygiene.

(65) (D) All of the above.

When providing mouth care, it is important to clean all parts of the mouth, including the tongue, the teeth, and the gums. Proper oral hygiene involves thorough cleaning of the entire mouth. The teeth need to be brushed to remove plaque and food particles. The gums should be gently cleaned to maintain gum health and prevent gum disease. The tongue also needs to be cleaned as it can harbor bacteria and food particles, and contribute to bad breath and oral health issues.

(66) (B) From front to back.

When perineal care is provided, the CNA should clean from front to back to prevent the entrance of bacteria from the rectum into the urinary tract.

(67) (B) From front to back.

Dry the patient from front to back to prevent the entrance of bacteria from the rectum into the urinary tract.

(68) (B) From front to back.

Dry the rectal area from front to back to prevent the entrance of bacteria from the rectum into the urinary tract.

(69) (A) Remove the footrests.

When a patient is transferred from the bed to a wheelchair, the footrests should be removed or folded up before the patient is assisted to stand.

(70) (C) Flat on the floor.

The patient should be assisted to a seated position with the feet flat on the floor. This helps to provide balance for the patient when they stand.

Test 8: Questions

(1) A CNA finds a 100-dollar bill beside a patient's bed. The patient is a 68-year-old man with severe Alzheimer's dementia. The CNA puts the money on the patient's bed where he can see it. The CNA acted with:

(A) Empathy.

(B) Compassion.

(C) Integrity.

(D) Safety.

(2) A certified CNA works in a big facility where people of different classes, races, and religions are treated. She ensures that everyone is treated with fairness and equality. Which principle of medical ethics guides her actions?

(A) Autonomy.

(B) Nonmaleficence.

(C) Justice.

(D) Fidelity.

(3) The medical record form that contains details about a patient's care, the methods, and frequency of care is referred to as the:

(A) Care plan.

(B) Flow sheet

(C) Nursing notes.

(D) Medical notes.

(4) A 54-year-old man comes to the emergency department with a fever and a cough productive of bloody sputum for a month. The patient is diagnosed with tuberculosis and placed in the isolation unit. What is the indication for the isolation of this patient?

(A) Privacy.

(B) Reduced stigma.

(C) Ensure adequate treatment.

(D) Prevent the spread of disease.

(5) What is an indication for the admission of a burn patient?

(A) Inhalational injury.

(B) Superficial burns.

(C) Burns in females.

(D) Burns in a young child.

(6) A 50-year-old man is brought to the emergency department with fever, diaphoresis, cough, and generalized weakness. Which of the following sites is not used to measure someone's temperature?

(A) Oral mucosa.

(B) Rectal mucosa.

(C) Armpit.

(D) Back.

(7) A five-year-old boy is brought to the emergency room with complaints of watery stool for the past three days. He is diagnosed with gastroenteritis with severe dehydration. Which of the following is a sign of dehydration in children?

(A) Swollen legs.

(B) Puffy face.

(C) Swollen abdomen.

(D) Sunken fontanelle.

(8) A CNA finds out that a patient has not had a bowel movement for the past four days. What is the next step that should be taken?

(A) Give the patient an enema.

(B) Give the patient a laxative.

(C) Perform a digital rectal examination.

(D) Inform the nurse about the change in the patient's bowel movement pattern.

(9) Which of the following is a role a CNA can perform in a patient's admission process?

(A) Measure the patient's vital signs.

(B) Perform a urinary catheterization.

(C) Perform a physical examination.

(D) Perform a medical screening.

(10) Which of the following investigations can be used to diagnose asthma?

(A) Chest X-ray.

(B) Electrocardiogram.

(C) Echocardiography.

(D) Spirometry.

(11) The hospice model of care is based on all of the following beliefs except:
(A) The dying person should not be separated from family members and other support systems.
(B) Dying is a normal and expected part of the life cycle.
(C) Hospice care seeks to help the person die with dignity.
(D) Pain is a normal and expected part of dying.

(12) In what circumstance will Medicare pay for the home healthcare cost of a client?
(A) If the client is chronically ill.
(B) If the client is financially constrained.
(C) If the client is homebound.
(D) If the client lives in a rural area.

(13) A 65-year-old patient has not passed stool in one day. The diagnosis of this patient is best described as:
(A) Constipation.
(B) Normal.
(C) Diarrhea.
(D) Loose stools.

(14) What is a risk factor for COPD?
(A) Smoking.
(B) Alcohol.
(C) Obesity.
(D) Hypertension.

(15) Which of the following is not a possible presentation of pressure ulcers?
(A) Skin erythema.
(B) Pain.
(C) Ulcers.
(D) No pulse.

(16) Which of the following is most important during mouth care?
(A) Rinse the mouth with sufficient water.
(B) Use diluted mouthwash.
(C) Use a hard toothbrush.
(D) Use different types of toothpaste.

(17) Which condition increases a patient's risk of a fracture or a fall?
(A) Diabetes.
(B) Dyslipidemia.
(C) Hypertension.
(D) Osteoporosis.

(18) A pureed diet is ordered for:
(A) Patients who can't chew or swallow solids.
(B) Newborns.
(C) Pregnant women.
(D) Adult patients.

(19) All of the following are consequences of untreated pain except:
(A) Sleep disturbances.
(B) Decreased mobility.
(C) Early healing.
(D) Change in appetite and weight.

(20) Mr. Coker dies from complications of heart and lung disease. Eight hours after his death, his muscles stiffen. This phenomenon is called:
(A) Solidification.
(B) Bone loss.
(C) Amputation.
(D) Rigor mortis.

(21) Which of the following is not a part of the stages of grief?
(A) Denial.
(B) Anger.
(C) Bargaining.
(D) Analogy.

(22) A 30-year-old man is brought to the emergency department because of an elated mood, excessive confidence, and grandiose delusions for the past two weeks. He spends money excessively and recently started gambling. What is the most likely diagnosis?
(A) Mania.
(B) Depression.
(C) Schizophrenia.
(D) Anxiety disorder.

(23) It is mealtime for a 60-year-old visually impaired patient. After she is served, what is the next best step for the CNA?
(A) Identify the location of food and utensils for the patient.
(B) Inform the patient to start eating.
(C) Drop the food off and go.
(D) Inform the patient to call when she finishes her meal.

(24) Which of the following can improve easy elimination in patients with chronic constipation?
(A) A high fiber diet.
(B) A low fiber diet.
(C) A high protein diet.
(D) A high sugar diet.

(25) A surgically created opening in the abdominal wall to help a patient with elimination is called:
(A) A drainage site.
(B) A stoma.
(C) An eliminator.
(D) A colon.

(26) A 56-year-old patient undergoes bowel resection due to gastric cancer. Which of the following is the best initial step after his surgery?
(A) Feed him a solid meal.
(B) Feed him a semisolid meal.
(C) Withhold enteral feeding for a month.
(D) Give him fluids and a liquid meal.

(27) Which of the following utensils helps to secure the plate on the tray?
(A) Gum tray.
(B) Plastic tray.
(C) Suction base.
(D) Both A and B.

(28) The biggest organ in the body is the:
(A) Eye.
(B) Brain.
(C) Skin.
(D) Liver.

(29) A 50-year-old male patient becomes aggressive with a CNA. What is the next best action for the CNA to take?
(A) Retreat to safety.
(B) Continue to try to provide care.
(C) Calm the patient down.
(D) Hold the patient until he calms down.

(30) Mrs. Samson is a 60-year-old patient who can walk without difficulty but needs help with balance. Which of the following devices is the best fit for the patient?
(A) Cane.
(B) Crutches.
(C) Wheelchair.
(D) Walker.

(31) A 65-year-old postmenopausal patient is being treated for osteoporosis. This condition can increase her risk of:
(A) Fractures.
(B) Bone cancer.
(C) Blindness.
(D) Osteoarthritis.

(32) A 64-year-old woman with diabetes mellitus develops recurrent chest pain. After investigations, she is told the chest pain is due to her heart not getting enough oxygen. This medical condition is referred to as:

(A) Angina.

(B) Heart failure.

(C) Pneumonia.

(D) Dyspnea.

(33) A 56-year-old woman with diabetes is rushed to the emergency room with a hyperosmolar hyperglycemic state, an acute diabetic emergency. Which of the following is a symptom most likely associated with the patient?

(A) Dehydration.

(B) Hemiplegia.

(C) Paraplegia.

(D) Rigidity.

(34) A 64-year-old patient is admitted to the ward and is managed for moderate persistent asthma. Which of the following should be within reach of the patient?

(A) A phone.

(B) An inhaler.

(C) Drugs.

(D) Water.

(35) All of the following are areas of concern to help a patient cope with losses and adjustment in nursing home placement except:

(A) Autonomy.

(B) Control.

(C) Exposure.

(D) Privacy.

(36) Who proposed a theory for the different levels of need an individual may encounter in order of priority?

(A) Sir Isaac Newton.

(B) Abraham Maslow.

(C) Albert Einstein.

(D) Albert Maslow.

(37) Mr. Stones, a 52-year-old accountant, feels unfilled in his career. How can a CNA help this client meet his self-actualization needs?

(A) Inform a colleague at Mr. Stones's work.

(B) Help Mr. Stones explore his values and interests and develop plans to pursue his goals.

(C) Ignore Mr. Stones as he will get more fulfilled with time.

(D) Report the situation to his family members.

(38) What is not a factor that promotes psychosocial well-being in older adults?

(A) A strong social support network.

(B) Exercise.

(C) Meaningful activities.

(D) Increased food consumption.

(39) All of the following are physical changes associated with aging except:

(A) Gradual loss of eyesight, hearing, smell, taste, and digestive functions.

(B) Renal dysfunction, such as urinary incontinence.

(C) Musculoskeletal decline.

(D) Optimal cardiovascular health.

(40) What is the primary concern for a stroke patient who has been in bed for two days?

(A) Pressure sores.

(B) Pulmonary embolism.

(C) Oral hygiene.

(D) All of the above.

(41) A CNA in the internal medicine department observes that a woman has a wound that refuses to heal after four weeks. What is the most likely reason?

(A) Diabetes.

(B) Heart failure.

(C) Hypertension.

(D) Brain tumor.

(42) A CNA struggles to remove a 45-year-old male patient's catheter. What should he do?
(A) Try again.
(B) Call for assistance.
(C) Use ultrasound guidance.
(D) Leave the catheter in place.

(43) Which of the following is not expected of a CNA who manages a patient with a femoral fracture?
(A) Assist with movement.
(B) Assist with bathing.
(C) Administer pain medication.
(D) All of the above.

(44) Which of the following is false about comfort for patients?
(A) It involves physical and emotional components.
(B) It differs from patient to patient.
(C) It involves only an emotional aspect.
(D) It involves patient monitoring.

(45) Which method is not useful to prevent falls?
(A) Use of bedrails.
(B) Feeding assistance.
(C) Bathing assistance
(D) Use of rugs.

(46) Which of the following is useful to reduce the risk of elopement?
(A) Sedatives.
(B) Color codes.
(C) Close monitoring.
(D) Both B and C.

(47) Which of the following is not an example of a comfort device?
(A) Cotton rings.
(B) Foot and knee rest.
(C) Pillows.
(D) Bedrails.

(48) The number of patients on a ward must be limited to prevent the spread of diseases like:

(A) Tuberculosis.

(B) Stroke.

(C) Fractures.

(D) Sickle cell.

(49) A man was stabbed in the left side of his chest. The knife stopped a few centimeters from his heart. What bony structure protected the heart?

(A) The myocardium.

(B) The ribs.

(C) The sternum.

(D) All of the above.

(50) A patient presents with anemia. Which of the following is the patient most likely to experience?

(A) Weakness.

(B) Swollen gums.

(C) Bleeding.

(D) Recurrent infection.

(51) Which bronchus is wider?

(A) The right bronchus.

(B) The left bronchus.

(C) Both are the same length.

(D) All of the above.

(52) The gastrointestinal system is made up of all of the following structures except:

(A) Teeth.

(B) Pharynx.

(C) Larynx.

(D) Salivary glands.

(53) A patient presents with Crohn's disease. What symptom is of concern to the CNA if the patient uses a bedpan?

(A) Cramps.

(B) Blood in the stool.

(C) Mucus.

(D) Blood in the urine.

(54) A 60-year-old man is admitted after a stroke. He has right-side paralysis. What side of the brain is most likely affected?

(A) The right side.

(B) The left side.

(C) All parts of the brain.

(D) The posterior side of the brain.

(55) A patient on the ward has Parkinson's disease. What are the possible complications to avoid in this patient?

(A) Falls.

(B) Depression.

(C) Immobility.

(D) All of the above.

(56) A CNA needs to turn a patient. He knows the following should be avoided:

(A) Falls.

(B) Patient lying on one arm.

(C) Waking up the patient.

(D) A and B.

(57) What is routinely used to clean the mouth?

(A) Toothbrush.

(B) Foam.

(C) Clothing.

(D) All of the above.

(58) Where should the toothpaste be applied when a patient's mouth is cleaned?
(A) To a moistened toothbrush.
(B) Inside the mouth.
(C) To a dry toothbrush.
(D) To the soft palate.

(59) What position should the patient be in while mouth care is provided?
(A) 140–180 degrees.
(B) 75–90 degrees.
(C) 10–30 degrees.
(D) 0–45 degrees.

(60) In what position must a patient be for the rectal area to be cleaned?
(A) Seated position.
(B) Upright position.
(C) On the side.
(D) Lithotomy position.

(61) What is a routine check that must be performed before perineal care is commenced?
(A) Ensure privacy with curtains or screens.
(B) Check the water temperature.
(C) Put on clean gloves
(D) All of the above.

(62) What is the primary purpose of a signaling device in a patient's room?
(A) For entertainment, such as watching TV or listening to music.
(B) To allow patients to adjust room temperature and lighting.
(C) To enable patients to call for assistance or alert staff to their needs.
(D) For monitoring the patient's vital signs remotely.

(63) A CNA wants to move a patient from the bed to a wheelchair. What is correct about this procedure?
(A) The patient does not need footwear when a transfer belt is used.
(B) It's okay for the patient to be barefoot during the procedure.
(C) The patient must put on shoes before the CNA helps him to stand.
(D) The client can only put on shoes after the CNA has helped him to stand.

(64) An example of a prearranged signal between a client and a CNA is:
(A) A countdown.
(B) Movement.
(C) Vulgar words.
(D) Offensive statements.

(65) A patient must be moved with a transfer belt. What is a safety precaution that must be observed?
(A) Lock the wheels on the wheelchair.
(B) Ensure the bed is at a safe level.
(C) Lock the bed wheels.
(D) All of the above.

(66) What is the correct position a patient should be in a wheelchair?
(A) With the hips against the wheelchair handle.
(B) With the waist against the back of the wheelchair.
(C) With the shoulders forward.
(D) With the hips against the back of the wheelchair.

(67) What should be used to wipe the bell of the stethoscope?
(A) Mercury.
(B) Alcohol.
(C) Iodine.
(D) All of the above.

(68) What artery is used to measure blood pressure?
(A) The radial artery.
(B) The ulnar artery.
(C) The brachial artery.
(D) The axillary artery.

(69) What is the first sound heard on deflation of the blood pressure cuff?
(A) Diastolic pressure.
(B) Systolic pressure.
(C) Fourth heart sound.
(D) Systemic pressure.

(70) What position should the stethoscope be in when blood pressure is measured?

(A) Bell/diaphragm – chest.

(B) Bell/diaphragm – elbow.

(C) Bell/diaphragm – forearm.

(D) Cuff – wrist.

Test 8: Answers and Explanations

(1) (C) Integrity.

Integrity is the quality of being trustworthy and honest. It also means strong moral principles, as demonstrated by this CNA.

(2) (C) Justice.

Justice is one of the core principles of medical ethics. It requires people to be treated equally and fairly without prejudice with respect to their race, color, class, social status, and religion. Autonomy is when healthcare workers allow patients to make decisions for their own health.

(3) (A) Care plan.

The care plan details a patient's management plan. It contains information about the management method, frequency of intervention, and medication doses.

(4) (D) Prevent the spread of disease.

Tuberculosis is a highly contagious airborne infection. The patient should be placed on respiratory isolation to prevent community spread.

(5) (A) Inhalational injury.

An inhalation injury is an indication for the admission of a patient with burns. Inhalational injuries are a serious concern as they can cause respiratory distress and other complications. These injuries occur when a person inhales hot gases, smoke, or toxic fumes during a fire, which can potentially damage the airways and lungs.

(6) (D) Back.

The thermometer is used to measure the surface or core body temperature. Body temperature can be measured at the armpit or mucosa. Mucous membranes that can be used to measure body temperature include the rectal and oral mucosa. Temperature is not measured objectively at the back.

(7) (D) Sunken fontanelle.

A sunken fontanelle is a sign of dehydration, particularly in children. Dehydration is caused by fluid loss through vomiting, gastroenteritis, and excessive sweating. Dehydration can be mild, moderate, or severe. It can be complicated by shock or acute kidney injury.

(8) (D) Inform the nurse about the change in the patient's bowel movement pattern.

When CNAs discover something out of the ordinary in a patient, they must escalate the matter to the nurse on duty. This patient may be constipated. It is the duty of the charge nurse to evaluate further and escalate as needed.

(9) (A) Measure the patient's vital signs.

During a patient's admission process, a CNA can measure the patient's vital signs. This includes checking and recording the patient's temperature, blood pressure, pulse rate, and respiratory rate.

(10) (D) Spirometry.

Spirometry is used to measure a patient's pulmonary function to diagnose asthma. Asthma is a chronic airway disease that is characterized by hyperresponsiveness. The obstruction is reversible with inhalers, other bronchodilators, and anti-inflammatory medications.

(11) (D) Pain is a normal and expected part of dying.

As part of comfort care, palliative treatment may be given to relieve uncomfortable symptoms. Pain medications may be administered, and dying should not necessarily involve pain.

(12) (C) If the client is homebound.

Medicare will pay for home healthcare costs only if the client is homebound. This means that the client requires significant effort to leave home and cannot leave without a great deal of assistance from another person.

(13) (B) Normal.

Normal bowel movements can occur up to once in three days. When a patient does not move their bowels in three days, constipation should be considered. When a patient moves their bowel three or more times a day, diarrhea should be evaluated and appropriately treated to prevent dehydration.

(14) (A) Smoking.

Smoking is a strong risk factor for COPD, which comprises emphysema and chronic bronchitis. Both are associated with progressive airway inflammation and damage. This leads to progressive cough, dyspnea, and eventual respiratory failure.

(15) (D) No pulse.

Pressure ulcers develop around bony prominences in the body, such as the sacrum, malleoli of the feet, etc. The first symptom of pressure ulcers is skin erythema. If left unattended, it progresses to ulcers, which can extend to deep tissues.

(16) (A) Rinse the mouth with sufficient water.

During mouth care, the mouth should be generously rinsed with sufficient water to ensure that all the debris is washed out. It helps to ensure no nidus for infection is left.

(17) (D) Osteoporosis.

Osteoporosis is a bone disease characterized by loss of bone mass. The remaining bone is soft and can fracture easily. Osteoporosis is seen frequently in elderly females and patients who often use steroids.

(18) (A) Patients who can't chew or swallow solids.

A pureed diet is prescribed for patients who recently had bowel surgeries, such as bariatric surgeries, gastric bypass, etc. The patients are started on pureed diets first and then gradually introduced to a solid diet.

(19) (C) Early healing.

Early healing is not a consequence of untreated pain. Instead, delayed healing, disturbances in sleep and sleep patterns, decreased mobility, variations in appetite and weight, reduced ability or desire to do routine activities, attend social functions and engage in interaction with others, and emotional effects such as depression are all consequences of untreated pain.

(20) (D) Rigor mortis.

Rigor mortis (stiffening of the muscles of the body) starts to develop about six to eight hours after death. It can be very difficult to reposition the body after rigor mortis occurs. Discoloration of the person's skin as a result of pooling of the blood also occurs.

(21) (D) Analogy.

The stages of grief are denial, anger, bargaining, depression, and acceptance. An analogy is not one of the stages.

(22) (A) Mania.

Mania is a mood disorder that is associated with an elated mood, excessive confidence, gambling, disorganization, and lavish spending. Patients often have grandiose delusions and believe they are very important people in society. The disorder may or may not be associated with psychotic symptoms.

(23) (A) Identify the location of food and utensils for the patient.

When a CNA helps a patient with a visual impairment who can eat on their own, the first thing to do is to show the patient the location of the food, plates, and cutlery. Once this is done, most patients with a visual impairment can eat on their own.

(24) (A) A high fiber diet.

Diets that are high in fiber are more easily eliminated from the gastrointestinal tract compared to diets that are low in fiber. To prevent constipation, patients are encouraged to eat food high in fiber. Patients are also encouraged to drink enough water and exercise regularly.

(25) (B) A stoma.

A stoma is a surgically created opening in the abdominal wall that connects the gastrointestinal tract to the external abdominal wall. It helps to redirect fecal matter to a tube connected to the abdominal wall.

(26) (D) Give him fluids and a liquid meal.

Fluids and liquid meals are the best initial meals for patients who recently underwent anastomosis.

(27) (C) Suction base.

A suction base is the utensil that helps to secure the plate on the tray. It is designed to provide stability and prevent the plate from sliding or moving around on the tray, which is particularly useful for individuals who may have difficulty with motor skills or coordination, such as those with certain disabilities or the elderly. The suction base attaches to the bottom of the plate and then firmly sticks to the tray, which creates a secure setup for eating.

(28) (C) Skin.

The largest organ in the body is the skin. It is made up of three major layers: the epidermis (the outermost layer), the dermis (the middle layer), and the subcutaneous layer (the innermost layer). The skin provides several functions, part of which is the protection of internal organs from diseases.

(29) (A) Retreat to safety.

When CNAs care for patients who are aggressive, violent, or disrespectful, the best next step is to temporarily withhold care and retreat to safety.

(30) (A) Cane.

A cane is a device used to facilitate easy mobility for patients who can move around but need support with balance. Canes are often used by the elderly who do not have musculoskeletal problems but are at risk of falls due to balance problems.

(31) (A) Fractures.

Osteoporosis is a demineralization of the bone that is common in postmenopausal women and individuals on steroids. Because the bones are soft and brittle, patients with osteoporosis are at risk of fractures.

(32) (A) Angina.

Angina is a medical condition that causes chest pain relieved by nitroglycerin. Angina occurs as a result of the coronary arteries being blocked by atherosclerotic plaques. This leads to a reduction in blood flow to the heart tissue and a reduced oxygen supply to the heart.

(33) (A) Dehydration.

Dehydration is a common presentation of hyperosmolar hyperglycemic state (HHS). The hyperosmolarity leads to dehydration (dry skin and mucosa).

(34) (B) An inhaler.

A patient with asthma should have their rescue inhaler as close to them as possible for use in emergencies.

(35) (C) Exposure.

Control, autonomy, and privacy are critical aspects of long-term care. Privacy, rather than exposure, is also an area of concern.

(36) (B) Abraham Maslow.

Abraham Maslow was a 20th-century American psychologist who developed a hierarchy of needs to explain human motivation in order of priority.

(37) (B) Help Mr. Stones explore his values and interests and develop plans to pursue his goals.

The CNA can help Mr. Stones explore his values and interests. The CNA can also help the client develop a plan to pursue his goals and dreams.

(38) (D) Increased food consumption.

Increased food consumption does promote improved psychosocial function in these patients.

(39) (D) Optimal cardiovascular health.

Optimal cardiovascular health is not a physical change associated with aging. Aging comes with a decline in various bodily functions, including cardiovascular health. As people age, they are more likely to experience issues such as increased blood pressure, reduced elasticity of blood vessels, and a higher risk of heart-related conditions. This is in contrast to the other options, which are common physical changes associated with aging.

(40) (D) All of the above.

A stroke patient who has been immobile for a long time can have a pulmonary embolism due to blood clots. Immobility can also cause pressure sores. Oral hygiene is also important in a patient like this to prevent bad odors, infections, and aspiration.

(41) (A) Diabetes.

Diabetes mellitus is characterized by slow wound healing as a result of nerve damage, impaired blood flow, and an increase in inflammation.

(42) (B) Call for assistance.

Sometimes, urinary catheters might prove difficult to remove. In such cases, a CNA should call for assistance. Nurses and doctors can then decide on the best way to remove the medical device.

(43) (C) Administer pain medication.

A CNA is not supposed to administer medications to patients. This is beyond the scope of a CNA's responsibilities.

(44) (C) It involves only an emotional aspect.

The statement that comfort for patients involves only an emotional aspect is false. Comfort for patients is a multifaceted concept that encompasses both physical and emotional components. Physical comfort can include managing pain, ensuring a comfortable position, and attending to basic needs like hunger and hygiene. Emotional comfort includes addressing psychological well-being, providing reassurance, and creating a calming environment.

(45) (D) Use of rugs.

The use of bedrails is important to prevent falls, especially at night. Assistance with meals and baths is also important. However, the use of rugs is a major risk factor for falls, especially in the elderly, because some rugs might fold or slip and cause the patient to trip.

(46) (D) Both B and C.

Color codes help everyone to know the patients and distinguish them. Close monitoring is also essential so that someone can always account for each patient at all times.

(47) (D) Bedrails.

Bedrails are not considered a comfort device. They are used for safety purposes, such as preventing patients from falling out of bed. Bedrails can also assist patients to reposition themselves in bed, but their main function is safety rather than comfort.

(48) (A) Tuberculosis.

One of the major risk factors for the spread of tuberculosis is overcrowding. This is why it's important to put too many people in a medical ward.

(49) (B) The ribs.

This patient's heart was protected by his ribs. The sternum is located more centrally, while the myocardium is the muscle directly on the heart.

(50) (A) Weakness.

Weakness is a common symptom of anemia. Anemia refers to the low level of red blood cells in the body. Weakness results because the body is not able to get an optimal level of oxygen. The brain is most affected by a lack of oxygen. Other vital organs like the heart and the kidneys are also affected.

(51) (A) The right bronchus.

The right bronchus is wider, shorter, and more vertical compared to the left bronchus. This anatomical difference is significant because it makes the right bronchus more prone to foreign object aspiration. If an object is inhaled and enters the bronchial tubes, it is more likely to lodge in the right bronchus due to its larger size and more direct path from the trachea.

(52) (C) Larynx.

The gastrointestinal system includes a series of organs involved in the digestion and absorption of food, but the larynx is not one of them. The larynx is part of the respiratory system and plays a key role in breathing, producing sound, and protecting the trachea against food aspiration.

(53) (B) Blood in the stool.

For a patient with Crohn's disease, the presence of blood in the stool is a symptom of concern when using a bedpan. Crohn's disease is a type of inflammatory bowel disease that can cause inflammation, ulcers, and bleeding in the digestive tract. Blood in the stool can indicate a worsening or complication of the disease, such as a significant flare-up or the development of ulcers in the intestines that are bleeding.

(54) (B) The left side.

A patient with right-side paralysis most likely had a left-sided stroke, because there is a crossing over of neurons.

(55) (D) All of the above.

Parkinson's disease can result in difficulty moving, falls, and depression because of the emotional trauma from the condition.

(56) (D) A and B.

Falls can be a risk factor for injury, fractures, loss of consciousness, and even death. Therefore, they must be prevented. A patient should also not lie on their arm, as this is an uncomfortable position and can result in pain.

(57) (A) Toothbrush.

A toothbrush is routinely used to clean the mouth. It is the standard tool for oral hygiene, and it is used to clean the teeth, gums, and the tongue. Toothbrushes help to remove food particles, plaque, and bacteria from the mouth, and thus maintain dental health and prevent oral diseases.

(58) (A) To a moistened toothbrush.

When cleaning a patient's mouth, toothpaste should be applied to a moistened toothbrush. This is the standard and effective method for oral hygiene. Moistening the toothbrush before applying toothpaste helps to soften the bristles and allows for better distribution of the toothpaste when brushing. It also makes the brushing experience more comfortable for the patient.

(59) (B) 75–90 degrees.

The patient should be sitting in an upright position at 75–90 degrees. This position is best to prevent aspiration into the lungs. It is also very comfortable for mouth care for both the CNA and the patient.

(60) (C) On the side.

To clean the rectal area, the patient is turned to the side and then cleaned from front to back.

(61) (D) All of the above.

All the steps listed are routine. A CNA should always ensure the privacy of patients, check that the water temperature is not too hot to cause burns, and wear clean gloves before the perineal area is washed.

(62) (C) To enable patients to call for assistance or alert staff to their needs.

A signaling device, often in the form of a call bell or button, is provided to patients in healthcare settings so they can easily alert the nursing staff or caregivers when they need help or assistance. This could be for a range of needs, from requiring help with using the restroom to urgent medical attention.

(63) (C) The patient must put on shoes before the CNA helps him to stand.

In the transfer of a patient from the bed to a wheelchair, the patient should be assisted to sit with his feet flat on the floor before he stands. This helps to provide balance. It's important that the patient wear shoes for additional stability.

(64) (A) A countdown.

A countdown is a good example of a prearranged signal between a CNA and a client to alert the patient of the exact time to stand.

(65) (D) All of the above.

In the movement of a patient with a transfer belt from the bed to the wheelchair, a CNA must ensure that all wheels on the wheelchair are locked, the bed is at a safe level, and all the bed wheels are also locked.

(66) (D) With the hips against the back of the wheelchair.

Appropriate positioning is critical when patients are moved with the transfer belt. The patient's hips should touch the back of the wheelchair.

(67) (B) Alcohol.

Alcohol has been shown to kill most bacteria and germs. Therefore, its use to clean the bell of the stethoscope will prevent the spread of infection.

(68) (C) The brachial artery.

The brachial artery is easily palpable and therefore is used to measure the blood pressure.

(69) (B) Systolic pressure.

The first sound heard on the deflation of the blood pressure cuff is the systolic pressure. It corresponds to the first heart sound.

(70) (B) Bell/diaphragm – elbow.

The position of the bell/diaphragm is on the elbow, where the heart sounds can be easily heard.

Access the Bonus Audiobook and Flash Cards!

Scan the QR code below with your phone and you will be given a link to Google Drive where you can download the audiobook and flash cards.

If the QR code does not work for you, please contact us at info@newstonetestprep.com and mention the title of this book.

Made in United States
North Haven, CT
10 November 2026

22097465R00167